Pharmacy Technician Tactics

A Strategic Approach to Pharmacy Technician Training

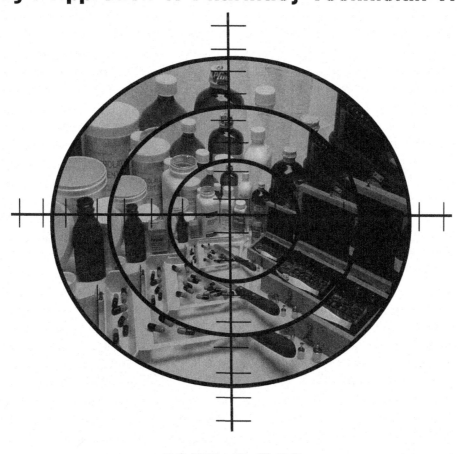

WILSON

ISBN 978-1-4675-3869-5

Pharmacy Technician Tactics: A Strategic Approach to Pharmacy Technician Training

Special thanks to Jennifer Herrington for her contribution of images found within the Mission 6 compounding studies. You are forever remembered and appreciated.

Acknowledgements

As the author and publisher of this text, I would like to give special thanks to those deserving individuals who have helped make this effort possible. To my husband, Darrell, you have given me unconditional love and support, time and the freedom to follow my dreams. To my sons, Cody, Tyler and Josh, thank you also for giving me a reason to follow those dreams. Without the four of you in my life this would all be worthless. To our parents, our brothers and sisters and other close friends and family: you have always been there when I called on you and to just say thank you would fall short on words, I'm afraid. To my best friend and helpmate, Silvia: Thank you for believing in me, backing me and encouraging me to go on even when things seemed impossible. I will be forever grateful to all of you for helping to make the last few years of my life, some of the best. This book is dedicated to each of you and to all the future students who will use it in an effort to find that new career path into the world of pharmacy. May God richly bless us each and every one.

Rhonda Wilson, CPhT

Tactics of Pharmacy Technician Training

In this study manual, you will be guided by tactics strategically planned to help you accomplish your mission of becoming a nationally certified pharmacy technician. Each area of training is announced with an icon or symbol to help you be more familiar with the expectations and training operations.

Mission Briefing: Before any military operation or assignment, a meeting or conference to announce or discuss actions and/or information needed to complete the mission is held in advance. This is done to alert everyone involved in the mission, the exact plans and purpose of the mission. In addition, any information that is needed to accomplish the mission at hand is distributed to those who need it. Each mission here in Pharmacy Technician Tactics is briefed with the appropriate objectives you will be striving to accomplish. The results of your accomplishments will be determined when you complete the mission debriefing at the close of each mission. The clipboard icon will help you find each list of mission objectives.

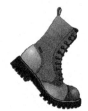

Military Drill and Ceremony: In our military branches, there are numerous opportunities to participate in parade drill and ceremony. The history of marching together in unison with precise movements, steps and the like goes way back in time. The actual act of moving as many troops as one unit was actually to strengthen the number. Alone a soldier in his/her own right may be a weak link but when together, each individual is upheld by the strength of peers. During my time of military service, I had the luxury (I call it that because not everyone got a chance take part) of participating in numerous parade drill and ceremony performances. In fact, it was probably what I enjoyed most about serving. How do that many individuals learn to work together as a team? How do they march together and move together in unison? Practice, practice and more practice. The cliché of "practice makes perfect" may be a cliché but a very obvious truth indeed! Throughout these individual missions, you will see the combat boot denoting **Drill Practice** activities. These suggested activities will strengthen what you have learned when used with the same practice makes perfect mentality.

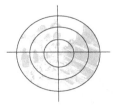

Target Terms: When a military firing mission has begun, there are generally specific targets of attack. Here in our strategic plan for your pharmacy technician training, target terms are located throughout each mission. These are important terms, definitions and acronyms that are needed to succeed in that particular mission. When listed throughout the mission training, the target terms will appear in **bold** text. During your study of each mission, you should come to obtain a full understanding of each of these Target Terms. Your knowledge of these terms will be tested when you complete the Mission Debriefing.

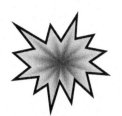

Math Blaster: When you see the explosion bubble, you are about to set out on a journey filled with math practice. There will be some math in every mission. Learning it this way does a couple of things. It prevents the entire math load from having to be learned at once in a single mission. Starting out you will be taking baby steps as if just beginning your training. As the missions continue toward the end of the training program, each step may build on the previous math learned and therefore continue the mission objectives needed to complete the training goal. There are many ways to do math but here in this training manual, there are some pretty interesting ways to accomplish your math goals. It is recommended to follow the instructions for the math so you will fully understand the process. Many steps can be left out once you are confident in your skills but as a rule, it is recommended to work out each step and write it down as instructed. These instructions will help you hone your math skills and be successful with pharmacy calculations. A good mantra to go by is "When in doubt, work it out!" Be ready for boot camp in math skills whenever you see the blast icon.

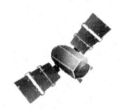

Reconnaissance Operations: Reconnaissance, by definition, is a military term used to describe the act of gathering intelligence or information to assist with the overall mission at hand. It is derived from the Old French language and means to explore or recognize. The military uses many forms of reconnaissance to gather information including air and ground observation, manned and unmanned aircraft and even satellites. In our strategic plan for your pharmacy technician training, there will be specific Recon Ops that are used for the same general purpose. These suggested extra-curricular exercises and field missions offer websites, books, articles or perhaps other types of information to strengthen what is offered here in this textbook. Each mission you encounter will have an area for suggested reading and research outside of the Pharmacy Technician Tactics training so that you can gather information relevant to your purpose. These recon missions allow you to obtain the most up to date information on specific subject areas. If such information had been included in print, it may change and therefore be out of date or invalid. Each time you see the satellite icon, you will know a **Recon Mission** is just around the corner.

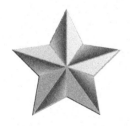

Mission Debriefings: Originating in military operations, mission debriefings are used to gather information from the mission participants regarding the accomplishments of that particular mission. Debriefings are a good evaluation tool to measure the successes of that mission based on the original mission objectives. If the mission was a failure, further discussion can determine the problems with the mission attempt and if necessary a regrouping and redeployment occurs. A member of the armed forces is generally eligible for promotion when a particular milestone has been met such as time in service, or successful duty performance. Awards or decorations are also given to those who have earned them for distinguished service. The military star icon alerts you to be advanced to the next mission upon completion of the mission debriefing.

Table of Contents

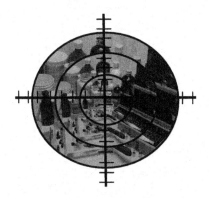

Mission 1:
Roles, Rules and
Regulations

Mission Objectives:

*To understand the roles and requirements of key players on the pharmacy team.
*To gain knowledge of the national certification process.
*To become familiar with the agencies who regulate the pharmacy industry.
*To understand the Federal laws that have affected our profession.
*To gain baseline knowledge of twelve of the most popular drugs on the market.
*To brush up on basic mathematical skills of rounding, decimals and percents.

Pharmacy technicians of today play a more important role in the work field than ever before. As the shortage of **pharmacists** takes its toile   on our nation, the role of the technician is expanding and ever changing. Most pharmacies have been utilizing pharmacy technicians, also known as **supportive personnel** for many years. Leaders in the pharmacy technician profession are striving to steer away from the term, supportive personnel, which is still used only in a minimal number of states. We prefer the more professional sound of the title, pharmacy technician.

As pharmacy technicians, we work alongside **registered pharmacists** who have at least 4 years and as many as 6 years or more of higher education. Those pharmacists with a **Doctor of Pharmacy** degree are known and recognized as **PharmDs** and have had to attend at least 6 or more years of higher education. Both pharmacists and PharmDs are usually required to have at least 20 hours of **continuing education** for every 2 years of practice though the requirements for pharmacists vary from state to state just as they do for pharmacy technicians. They have endured long, long hours of studying and working to get where they are.

In the pharmacy arena, you are generally encouraged to follow the **chain of command**. Since this chain can vary from employer to employer, we will take a look at some common levels of leadership you may encounter. Pharmacy technicians may be on various levels of knowledge and/or training and therefore a structure within the technician rank is not uncommon. Technicians may or may not have had formal training depending solely on the past and present requirements of that particular state. Some pharmacies may refer to their technician rank as levels. For instance, Level I, Level II or Level III technicians. Others may refer to them as technicians, lead technicians or even technician supervisors.

Many years ago, "druggists" may have been able to be apprenticed into their positions. This means that they worked a certain number of required years under another "druggist" to learn all there was to know before being allowed to practice on his/her own. Now, pharmacists, whether they are Registered Pharmacists (RPh) or Doctors of Pharmacy (PharmD), do require formal education and plenty of it. Registered pharmacists have had 3 to 5 years of higher education and have earned at minimum a Bachelor's Degree in Pharmacy. The newer generation of pharmacists has had to attend as much as 6 and now 7 required years of higher education to earn that same level of learning.

Pharmacies not only have a common rank structure for their technician employees, there will also be a rank structure for pharmacists as well. **Staff pharmacists** take care of the general duties of the pharmacist. **Shift supervisors** will be in charge of their entire shift of staff including both staff pharmacists and technicians. The **Pharmacist-in-Charge** or **PIC** is responsible for all staff and the daily operations of the pharmacy. There may be more than one PIC due to the rotation of duty days and non duty days. The **pharmacy manager** will be the overall leader of a particular pharmacy. (Sometimes the pharmacy manager and the PIC will be the same person) If the pharmacy is part of a chain or corporation, there will be a **district manager** over several stores within the area. As we continue up the ladder, there will likely be a **regional manager** to whom all the district managers report. At the top of the leadership chain, there will be a **corporate manager**.

Ranks of Pharmacy Leadership

Corporate Manager
Regional Manager
District Manager
Pharmacy Manager
Pharmacist-in-Charge
Shift Supervisor
Staff Pharmacists
Lead Technicians/Technician Supervisors
Other levels of technician personnel

Hopefully this gives you a more formidable idea of the infrastructure of leadership within the pharmacy. Remember that each particular state, region, district, chain or other jurisdiction may have various titles for each of these positions. Once on the job, it will not be long before you know all the ranks of your new employer and coworkers.

Our paths cross those of many others in the medical arena on a daily basis and we always need to function within the limited scope of our profession's practice. We should be aware of our boundaries and stay within them. There are very specific laws as to how technicians may assist in every aspect of pharmacy. Performing tasks that are not legally allowed may constitute practicing pharmacy without a license, which is punishable by law.

Those in the medical arena whose paths we may cross can be separated into two major categories…those who can prescribe medications and those who cannot. Listed below are the acronyms and key word descriptions of those who can and cannot prescribe medications.

Who can Prescribe Medications: Medications:

MD – Doctor of Medicine, Medical Doctor

DO – Doctor of Osteopathy

DDS – Dentist

PDOC – Psychiatrist

PA – Physician's Assistant

FNP – Family Nurse Practitioner

CNM – Certified Nurse Midwife

DPM – Podiatrist

OD – Optometrist

OPH – Opthalmologist

PharmD – Doctor of Pharmacy

Who cannot Prescribe

DC - Chiropractor

PsyD - Psychologist

RD - Dietician

RN – Registered Nurse

LPN – Licensed Practical Nurse

RPh - Pharmacist (Registered)

OT – Occupational Therapist

PT - Physical Therapist

ST – Speech Therapist

Although, at this time, **national certification** is not required by some states, it is an aspect of the profession that is looked highly upon by many employers. As the role of the technician advances, employers and pharmacists alike will desire the technician who has proven himself through standardized levels of training and competency exams over one who has not done so.

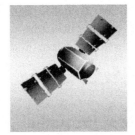

Recon Mission 1:

There are currently two organizations that are offering competency exams to render the credential of national certification of pharmacy technicians. They and their website addresses are as follows:

- **The Pharmacy Technician Certification Board (PTCB)** offers the Pharmacy Technician Certification Exam (PTCE) (www.ptcb.org)
- **National Healthcareer Association (NHA)** offers the Exam for the Certification of Pharmacy Technicians (ExCPT) (www.nhanow.com)

You will want to visit those websites and learn more about these organizations and the process by which you can become nationally certified as a pharmacy technician. Each organization has their own prerequisites and limitations for those who can apply for the exam process as well as their own listings for exam content and formatting. Both groups now offer a pass/fail notification on test day as well as various days and times for testing at numerous locations. Taking and passing either competency exam will give the same credentialing of nationally certified pharmacy technician or **CPhT**.

_____

Though state law varies from state to state across the nation most all of the states do have/require some form of **registration** or **licensure** for every technician employed in the state. Registration is generally obtained by submitting a completed written application along with paying a fee to the **State Board of Pharmacy (SBOP)**. Typically the registration must be renewed annually and the pharmacy board requires notification in writing of change of employment or change of address.

The requirements for pharmacy technicians in your state can be found by contacting the board directly by mail, phone or online. Regulations will vary from one state to another so never assume that just because one state has certain requirements that others will have the same requirements. You should always follow the standards that are accepted/required in the state where you live and work.

The registration or licensure requirement is a big step for technicians. Although it may seem to some as just another fee, it says something. It says that you are a pharmacy technician, duly registered by your State Board of Pharmacy to be employed. It is a start to better regulations, professional recognition and greater compensation for the job you perform as a pharmacy technician.

In addition to regulating the role of the pharmacy technician, each individual Board of Pharmacy is responsible for overseeing the entire practice of pharmacy within its respective state. This includes regulation of licensure, responsibilities, and requirements for pharmacists, technicians, other medical professionals who are involved in dispensing medications and also the facilities in which these medications are dispensed.

Additionally, the individual state boards govern the policies and procedures for dispensing functions and control of inventory. The ultimate goal of the individual boards is to ensure that quality pharmacy practice is provided for the health of the public in a safe, accurate and effective manner.

In addition to the SBOP, there are other agencies involved in the regulation and governance of pharmacy practice and all that it entails.

The **National Association of Boards of Pharmacy (NABP)** is a professional organization that represents each of the fifty state boards, boards in the outer lying territories of the United States and those in several other countries. The mission of NABP is to assist its member boards and jurisdictions in developing uniform standards and also to helping to get those standards implemented and enforced. The purpose of this association is to promote protection of the public's health. Though this organization does not make the laws, which must be done by the individual state boards, they do make suggestions for both laws and regulations for the practice of pharmacy. There is further information about **NABP** and links to each state's Board of Pharmacy websites located at www.nabp.net .

Joint Commission on Accreditation of Healthcare Organizations (JCAHO), otherwise known as "Jayco", is also involved in setting standards. As a matter of fact, JCAHO is known for accrediting around 88% of health care organizations including around 19,000 hospitals, long term care facilities, laboratories and clinics through evaluations and inspections. Generally, their facility inspections fall on triennial years, though they can visit an accredited facility at any time and can do so unannounced.

It is an independent, non-profit group, which predominates standards setting in the health care field. This organization strives to improve both quality and safety of healthcare provided to the public domain. JCAHO standardizes the performance improvement and quality assurance of institutions all over the country that are accredited organizations. Feel free to learn more at www.jcaho.org.

The **Food and Drug Administration (FDA)** meets its mission by creating standards as well. This government organization establishes and enforces high product standards and other regulations and requirements as authorized and mandated by the **Federal Food, Drug and Cosmetic Act.** The FDA does not regulate the practice of pharmacy but it does regulate sales and distribution practices of pharmacy and providers. The FDA is also the organization responsible for approving food, drugs and cosmetics for market as well as recalling those products that have been deemed unsafe for consumers.

The Food and Drug Administration oversees the **Med Watch** program. This program is a voluntary reporting program where information is reported regarding adverse events. An event should be reported to the FDA whether or not it is known if a drug or other medical device was the cause of the event. Located at www.fda.gov is much more information regarding what the Food and Drug Administration does oversee.

The **DEA** or **Drug Enforcement Administration** is a division of another government agency known as the **Department of Justice.** The DEA is responsible to enforce laws regarding controlled substances within the medical field. It also does everything possible to bring to justice any individuals or members of organizations involved in growth, manufacture and distribution of illicit drugs in the United States and its territories.

The *DEA* also supports programs aimed at reducing the availability of those illicit substances in the domestic and international markets as well. www.dea.gov is where more information is available on the regulations enforced by this administration including the **Controlled Substances Act of 1970.** This group of laws enacted over four decades ago separates controlled substances into schedules I through V based on their potential for danger and abuse by the public.

One last government organization, **The Centers for Medicare and Medicaid Services (CMS),** formerly known as HCFA administers the **Medicare** program. This program is primarily for seniors who have reached the age of 65 but may also cover those individuals who have become disabled before they reach 65. There are several parts to the Medicare program.

Part A is available at no charge to eligible individuals and covers hospital and inpatient services. **Part B** is available to eligible patients willing to pay the standard monthly premium and it covers the majority of outpatient and clinic services. **Part D** covers prescription drugs for those eligible patients who have chosen to enroll and pay a monthly premium into a **Prescription Drug Plan (PDP).**

In order to be eligible for Part D enrollment, an individual MUST have either Part A OR Part B. They need not have both to enroll into a Part D PDP. Medicare Part C is often referred to as the Medicare Advantage program and in order to enroll in Part C, an individual MUST have BOTH Parts A and B. Though new Medicare eligible patients have a seven month window (The three months before and after and including their 65th birth month)to enroll in Medicare and the various parts thereof, the annual open enrollment period for Parts C and D lasts about six weeks and comes at the end of each year with dates set by CMS.

The Centers for Medicare and Medicaid Services (CMS) partners with individual states to administer the **Medicaid** program. State Medicaid programs have inclusion for individuals who meet income and resource restrictions for the Aged, Blind and Disabled. They also have programs for Pregnant Women and Children ages 18 and under. If a patient is Medicare eligible AND Medicaid eligible and are enrolled in both, we refer to those individuals as having "dual eligibility". In such cases, usually the state Medicaid division will "pay" the premiums for that patient's Medicare premiums for Part B and D coverage.

In addition, the Social Security Administration will pay the part D premiums for those individuals who may be above income and resource limits for Medicaid but are still below a certain percentage of the Federal Poverty Level as determined on an annual basis. These individuals qualify for "extra help" from Social Security and receive a Low Income Subsidy(LIS) benefit. The benefit may range from 25% to 100% of the individual's premium amount paid on their behalf.

If a family does not meet the stringent restrictions for income and resources to be eligible for Medicaid, they may qualify for benefits through the **State Children's Health Insurance Program (SCHIP)**. Though initially intended for children 18 and under, the coverage has expanded in some states to include the parents of those children.

In addition to all of the above, CMS standardizes and enforces the **Health Insurance Portability and Accountability Act of 1996 (HIPAA)**. CMS oversees spending nearly 25 percent of all Federal Government dollars to ensure that as many American men, women and children as possible, who are eligible, have health insurance coverage.

Though there have been numerous laws over the years and even amendments to those laws passed, there are some major laws that stand out as an integral part of shaping the practice of pharmacy. You should familiarize yourself with these laws listed below and take note of their chronology. If given a particular practical situation, be able to determine which of the laws is being followed, abused or neglected.

Major Federal Pharmacy Laws

1906 – Federal Food and Drug Act – One of the first laws enacted to prevent the sale of inaccurately labeled drugs. It required manufacturers to put only truthful information on product labels.

1914 – Harrison Narcotic Act – The first of several attempts to control drug trafficking in the US. This law required a prescription in order to obtain opium.

1938 – Food, Drug and Cosmetic Act – Enacted to fill gaps in the earlier law including cosmetics. It prohibited misbranding or adulteration of drugs. There were also new labeling requirements. "Warning: May be habit forming" had to be on all controlled substances. Package inserts and directions to the consumer for use were also required.

1951 -Durham-Humphrey Amendment- This change increased requirements for drug manufacturers and separated legend drugs (prescription only) from non-legend drugs (otc). It also required "Caution: Federal law prohibits dispensing without a prescription" on all legend drugs. This caution is sometimes replaced with the "Rx only" message.

1962- Kefauver-Harris Amendments – This change attempted to ensure the safety and effectiveness of all new drugs on the market and Good Manufacturing Practices were put into place.

1970 – Controlled Substances Act – This law among other things is most known for setting ground rules for controlled drugs and their distribution. It separated them into the five schedules based on their potential for abuse.

1970- Poison Prevention Act – Required (with few exceptions) childproof caps on all medications dispensed in an outpatient setting. A patient or physician can make a request for non-safety caps. Some medications are not feasibly childproofed and are exempted. One, in particular, is nitroglycerin. This medication should not be dispensed in a childproof container. It is indicated for angina (chest pain) and must be kept in its original glass container which includes a non-safety cap.

1983- Orphan Drug Act – This law allowed companies to bypass the time requirements of new drug testing so that persons with rare diseases or terminal illnesses such as cancers would have access to new "hopeful" medications.

1987 Prescription Drug Marketing Act – This law required the same controls on drugs for animals to be ordered by a licensed veterinarian and to have similar labeling requirements.

1990 Omnibus Budget Reconciliation Act (OBRA) – This law, which dealt primarily with Medicare/Medicaid reimbursement, required pharmacies to make an offer of counsel by a pharmacist to all persons covered under Medicare/Medicaid for new prescriptions.

1996- Health Insurance Portability and Accountability Act- Provided continuance of health insurance even when changing employers. It also has had several parts that have taken effect at different stages. The area that affected the pharmacy field most of all is that concerning patient privacy that took effect April 15, 2003. This law was implemented and is enforced by CMS.

1997- FDA Modernization Act – Among other things, this made provisions for compounding of medications on-site in the pharmacy that were not commercially available at the time.

2005 – Combat Methamphetamine Epidemic Act- This law required all products containing pseudoephedrine to be moved behind the pharmacy counter. Though these products could still be bought without a prescription, all purchases were now accounted for by requiring a picture ID as well as a recorded signature. Note that several states including Oregon, Mississippi and Missouri have since made those same products containing the pseudoephedrine a scheduled 3 controlled substance. This change has decreased the numbers of meth labs significantly enough to have many other states looking into passing similar laws.

Though you will study individual practice settings more closely in the coming chapters, we will take a look at some general facts that affect all technicians and cross over to all areas of pharmacy practice.

Ratio laws vary from state to state. Some states do not even have a pharmacist to technician ratio; others have as high as four to one ratio. The majority of boards allow only two pharmacy technicians on duty performing work related to the dispensing of medications for each pharmacist. This doesn't mean that only two techs can be employed, or that only two can be on duty at the same time. Other technicians performing non-dispensing duties such as filing prescriptions for long term storage, delivery, and general record keeping do not have to be counted in this two-to-one ratio of technicians to pharmacists.

Pharmacist-to-technician ratio is the set number of technicians that can be supervised by a pharmacist according to the law. The most common ratio across the nation is two technicians to one pharmacist.

The regulations usually state that every person serving as a pharmacy technician must wear a **nametag,** while on duty, identifying him/herself as such. In addition, when communicating by telephone to patients, customers, or other medical personnel, a technician must promptly identify him/herself as such. The last thing that we want to do as profession technicians is to give a false impression of our rank in the pharmacy.

Although the practice of pharmacy, in most cases, allows the use of technicians, the pharmacist-in-charge (PIC) should see that the technician is properly trained for the job tasks he/she performs. The technician should always be working under the direct supervision of a pharmacist. With that being said, most pharmacies have policies in place that prohibit technicians being in a pharmacy dispensing area without a pharmacist present.

The duties performed by the tech should be consistent with the training and experience they have received and the laws set forth by the State Board of Pharmacy. In this case, knowledge is power. The broader the knowledge base is, the more responsibility a technician can undertake, and a higher pay is generally given to compensate.

Even though all technicians working for the same employer might have different levels of experience and training, here are some general areas that technicians share the responsibility with others in their profession.

*The pharmacy area should be maintained in an orderly, sanitary condition.

*Drug storage areas should be kept free of dust, dirt and grime.

*Countertop, shelving and floor spaces should be kept free of clutter and other items which could interfere with the dispensing process.

*Expired medications should be promptly removed from stock and handled accordingly because it is unlawful for a pharmacy to sell or dispense expired pharmaceuticals whether or not it was intentional.

*All pharmacy personnel share the responsibility of confidentiality issues. Information should not be repeated or released unless authorization has been given.

Pharmacy technicians in different work settings may be doing totally different jobs while sharing the same profession. The two main work settings are ambulatory care and institutional pharmacy. Ambulatory care, often called retail or outpatient pharmacy is a challenging, yet rewarding experience. These technicians are in constant contact with the patients that they serve. The typical settings range from small independent retail pharmacies to larger chain pharmacies. Even techs that are employed in government facilities like the VA hospitals, Indian Health Service facilities and military installations all fit into this outpatient category.

The majority of the duties in this line of work revolve around the dispensing process, inventory and purchasing, third party billing and reconciliation, and customer service. Although a technician may receive written prescriptions, in most states, a tech cannot receive new prescriptions by oral communication. Only a pharmacist may receive incoming prescriptions by telephone or verbal order. A pharmacy technician is not allowed to interpret orders to other individuals in transferring or providing a verbal copy to another pharmacy.

Although, technicians can perform a majority of the dispensing functions, including typing labels and filling prescriptions, it is the pharmacist that is responsible for verification of the finished product. A technician is NOT allowed to **counsel** a patient concerning his/her medicines. Much of the information given during counseling requires professional judgment, for which a technician is not qualified to provide.

Though state law prohibits technicians from counseling patients, often qualified technicians can give some educational information such as diabetic home monitoring help. Some pharmacies have separate personnel or clerks to operate the cash register, but in smaller pharmacies technicians do a wide variety of tasks, including running the cash register and billing statements.

Pharmacy technicians working in a totally different environment are those known as institutional pharmacy technicians. A technician working in the hospital setting may be responsible for daily dose picking for the unit-dose cart fill and preparation of intravenous admixtures. In addition, technicians are also allowed by law to assist the pharmacist in other compounding. It is the responsibility of the pharmacist to train and monitor the technician. A pharmacy technician's compounding duties should be consistent with the training he/she has received in this field.

Some larger inpatient facilities now have automated distribution systems (ADS) or electronic counting machines. These may be filled/stocked/replenished by technicians or other qualified personnel. In the institutional setting the duty of monthly unit inspections most always falls on the technician staff. Inspections would include checking for expired medications, proper storage, and other issues. If problems or concerns were found, they would be reported to a pharmacist for follow-up.

Inventory and purchasing are two areas where the technician can play a major role. The pharmacist must again verify all technician work to assure accuracy; however, in some states duly qualified and trained technicians are responsible for tech-check-tech. Such instances include refilling unit-dose cart fill medications and stocking medication distribution systems. This exception of tech-check-tech would never include final verification of a prescription prior to being dispensed to the patient.

Direct patient care is becoming more the norm in the field of pharmacy. Techs in different settings are involved in direct patient care in various ways. Retail and outpatient pharmacy technicians interact with patients and their family members on a regular basis, from phone conversations, handling insurance situations, to assisting in over-the-counter items. Hospital and inpatient pharmacy technicians do not have the one-on-one contact patient contact.

The innovative roles that are becoming the standard for many techs in the work setting are involved in direct patient care in another aspect. Since the technicians are handling more of the dispensing process, the pharmacists' time is freed up for other things. Retail pharmacists are able to provide better counseling to improve patient compliance, safety and accuracy. Hospital pharmacists are often making rounds with physicians to play a more clinical role in direct patient care.

Math Blaster

Starting off with some very basic math skills can work into some very complicated pharmacy calculations. If the basics are understood and one can work miracles with small numbers that are non-pharmacy related, it will help to see past the confusion of adding pharmacy information into the problems.

Place Value

Every digit in a number has place value. The numbers to the left of a decimal point are whole numbers and those to the right of a decimal point are a fraction of a whole number. Looking at the number below, take note to the place value of each digit given.

$$12345.6789$$

1	2	3	4	5	.	6	7	8	9
ten-thousands	thousands	hundreds	tens	ones	decimal point	tenths	hundredths	thousandths	ten-thousandths

With that being said, the rule of rounding is based on the number "5". The place value of numbers has plenty to do with rounding. If asked to round off a number to a specific place value, for instance, to the nearest tenth or thousandth, that means that particular place value needs to be kept and everything else to the right of that place value needs to be discarded. The rounded value of the place value kept is determined by the value of the number just to the right of that particular place.

If rounding to the nearest whole number or "ones" then the determining number would be the in the "tenths" place. If rounding to the nearest hundredth then the determining number would be in the thousandths place. Using that determining number, if it is 5 or greater, the place value you are keeping would be rounded up or if it is 4 or less, the place value you are keeping would remain unchanged and finally all numbers to the right of that kept number would be discarded.

Decimals and Percents

A decimal point is but a simple thing; however, it can greatly affect the outcome of a calculation. The reason why is that and error by marking a decimal point to the right or to the left of where it actually should be can change the numerical value by ten times, a hundred times or even a thousand times or more. Where pharmacy calculations are concerned, having a good understanding of the concept of decimals and percents is a must!

Percent values, are as equally important for attention to detail. The word "percent" actually explains a lot. "Cent" is the root meaning hundred so percent or per hundred is what is being spelled out with a percent. For instance, if 88% of pharmacy patients at a particular pharmacy are NOT allergic to penicillin that means that 88 patients of every hundred patients counted are not allergic to penicillin.

With that being said, most calculators have a percent key (%) and it can become a new best friend or worst enemy when running calculations. One can multiply and divide with it and it will make things a good bit simpler. The important thing to remember when using the % key on the calculator is to not follow it with the "=" sign. For instance, if the following was performed on a calculator, it would look something like this.....

100 x 88% $\longrightarrow$ 88

If the % was followed by the = sign it changes the number drastically though. It would look something like this which is incorrect for what would be sought.

100 x 88% = $\longrightarrow$ 8800

Just don't get into a habit of hitting = after the % signs are used and it should be fine. Confidence will come in math skills as practice continues training program and it will become second nature.

From Decimal to Percent

The transition from a decimal to a percent can be done several ways. Considering the fact that these numerous ways end up with the same answer, The focus will be on what is probably the easiest way of doing it: Simply moving the decimal point to the right or to the left.

When going from a decimal to a percent value, the mathematical process involves multiplying by the number 100. However, in doing that, the decimal point simply moves two places to the right. When going from a percent to a decimal value, it involves dividing by that number 100 and doing so results in the decimal point being two places to the left. The easiest way is to remember your alphabet and the letters "D" and "P".

D comes before P in the alphabet so set them up likewise…. Follow along to the numbers to gain a better perspective.

D P

Now, imagine that the decimal point is just to the left of the "D" as it will be when you are working with a number in "decimal point" value. Then move it two places to the right to arrive at that same number but now in percent form because the decimal has been moved to percent value. Imagine it something like this…

.D P ⟶ D P. ⟶ %

0.88 ⟶ 88. ⟶ 88%

At this point, discard the decimal and add the percent sign because the number is now in percent form.

14

From Percent to Decimal

This process is reversed from the previous instructions. D still comes before P in the alphabet so set them up likewise.... Follow along to the numbers to gain a better perspective.

D P

Now, imagine that percent sign has been discarded and the decimal point is just to the right of the "P" as it will be when you are working with a number in "percent" value. Then move it two places to the left to arrive at that same number but now in decimal form because the decimal has been moved to decimal value. Imagine it something like this...

.D P   ←—   D P.   ←—   %

0.88   ←—   88.   ←—   88%

Taking what has been learned through these instructions, work through the drill practice to increase confidence in these basic skills.

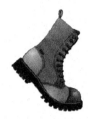

Drill Practice

Complete the following then check yourself in the rear of the textbook.

Round the following numbers to:

the nearest whole number

1. 1.2
2. 3.7
3. 6.2
4. 7.9

the nearest tenth.

5. 6.87
6. 3.52
7. 2.09
8. 78.42

the nearest hundredth.

9. 71.247
10. 2.682
11. 58.679
12. 101.097

the nearest thousandth.

13. 25.6428
14. 218.8693
15. 1049.0309
16. 12.0071

Change the following numbers from decimal value to percent form:

17. 0.32
18. 0.74
19. 0.08
20. 0.81

21. 0.4
22. 0.025
23. 0.8
24. 0.0475

Change the following numbers from percent form to decimal value:

25. 96%
26. 3.27%
27. 47.8%
28. 56%

29. 2%
30. 0.8%
31. 74%
32. 2.87%

16

Drug Training Chapter One

Brand Name	Generic Name	Drug Classification	Primary Indication	Side effects, Warnings, Other
Levaquin	Levofloxacin	Fluroquinolone AntiBacterial Agent	treat various types of infection	Fluoroquinolones are associated with an increased risk of tendinitis and tendon rupture, Should not be used in patients less than 18 years
Zyloprim	Allopurinol	Anti-Gout	Reduce uric acid level	Skin rash, diarrhea, nausea
Cardizem CD	Diltiazem CD	Calcium Channel Blocker	Hypertension	Lower limb edema, bradycardia, dizziness, fatigue, cough
Seroquel	Quetiapine	Anti- Psychotic Agent	Schizophrenia, BiPolar disorder	Warning: Increased mortality in elderly patients with dementia-related psychosis; somnolence, dizziness, dry mouth, constipation, weight gain and dyspepsia
Lortab, Lorcet, Vicodin	Hydrocodone/ Acetaminophen	C III Opioid Analgesic	Moderate to Moderately Severe Pain	Drowsiness, Dizziness,Lethargy, Nausea & Vomiting, Constipation
Xanax	Alprazolam	C IV Benzodiazepine	Anxiety disorder	Drowsiness, Light-headedness, Dry-mouth
Coumadin	Warfarin	Anti-Coagulant	Prophylaxis treatment of venous thrombosis and pulmonary embolism.	Can cause major or fatal bleeding, parasthesia, pain, dizziness. Vitamin K is the reversal drug used for warfarin blood levels that need to be lowered.
Eskalith	Lithium Carbonate	Anti-Psychotic Agent	Manic episodes of manic-depressive illness	Fine hand tremor, polyuria, mild thirst, transient and mild nausea
Amoxil	Amoxicillin	Pencillin Derivative Antibiotic	Broad spectrum Antibacterial	Candidiasis, GI upset, may cause reduced effectiveness of contraceptives

Brand Name	Generic Name	Drug Classification	Primary Indication	Side effects, Warnings, Other
Singulair	Montelukast	Leukotriene Receptor Antagonist	Prophylaxis/ Chronic treatment of Asthma, Allergic Rhinitis, Exercise Induced Broncho-constriction	Upper respiratory symptoms and infections, fever, headache, pharyngitis, cough, abdominal pain, diarrhea
Prilosec	Omeprazole	Proton-Pump Inhibitor	Duodenal or Gastric Ulcers, (GERD) Gastro-esophageal Reflux Disease	Headache, abdominal pain, nausea and vomiting, diarrhea and flatulence
Motrin	Ibuprofen	NSAID	Mild to Moderate pain and inflammation	May increase risk of serious cardiovascular events which can be fatal. May also cause GI bleeding, nausea, and other abdominal disturbances.

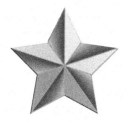

Mission 1 Debriefing

Answer the following questions in assessment of the lessons learned in Mission 1. For best results, repeat the exercise until no questions are missed then move on to the next mission.

1. Which of the following would typically be required to register with the State Board of Pharmacy?
   a) Pay an annual fee
   b) Give notice of change in address or employment
   c) Submit an application
   d) Renew annually
   e) all of these

2. The drug called allopurinol is indicated for use in treating _____.
   a) mild to moderate pain
   b) schizophrenia
   c) gout
   d) infection

3. A small chain pharmacy employs only one pharmacist per shift. The company's policy states that no one can be in the dispensing area without a pharmacist. A technician has asked the Pharmacist in Charge could she work through lunch and get off an hour early. He agrees. What should the technician do while the pharmacist is out to lunch?
   a) Front the OTC area and clean up the patient waiting area
   b) Return meds to the pharmacy's inventory that were not picked up by the patients.
   c) Make calls to insurance companies to catch up on "problem" claims
   d) Restock vials and caps for the evening shift

4. Which of these medications is a broad spectrum antibacterial agent?
   a) Cardizem CD
   b) Seroquel
   c) Eskalith
   d) Amoxil

5. Who cannot carry the responsibility of prescribing medications?
   a) Doctor of Pharmacy
   b) Family Nurse Practitioner
   c) Licensed Practical Nurse
   d) Physician's Assistant
   e) Registered Pharmacist
   f) A, B, D and F only
   g) C and E only
   h) All of these

6. Approximately how much of all Federal Government dollars are spent on health insurance so programs such as Medicare, Medicaid and CHIPS can be available to those who qualify.
   a) 10%
   b) 15%
   c) 20%
   d) 25%

7. The drug hydrocodone/acetaminophen is a Class _____ controlled substance.
   a) 2
   c) 4
   b) 3
   d) 5

8. A registered pharmacist cannot verify a technician's work for final dispensing to a patient.
   a) True
   b) False

9. Most individual state boards of pharmacy now require some form of _____ or _____ to practice as a technician.
   a) Certification
   c) licensure
   b) registration
   d) education

10. Which of the following drugs is classified as an NSAID?
    a) ibuprofen
    c) omeprazole
    b) montelukast
    d) hydrocodone/acetaminophen

11. The Drug Enforcement Agency is responsible for guarding misuse of both prescription related controlled drugs as well as those illicit street drugs.
    a) True
    b) False

12. The most common ratio of technicians to pharmacists across the nation is _____.
    a) 2:1
    c) 4:1
    b) 3:1
    d) most states do not have ratio laws

13. It is unlawful for a pharmacy to sell expired merchandise knowingly OR unknowingly to their patients.
    a) True
    b) False

14. What is the group of laws enforced by the DEA responsible for separating drugs into schedules I through V based on their potential for harm or abuse known as?
    a) Harrison Narcotic Act of 1914
    b) Kefauver-Harris Amendment 1962
    c) Controlled Substances Act of 1970
    d) Durham-Humphrey Amendment of 1951

15. The drug Levaquin is classified as a(n)_____.
    a) antiasthmatic
    c) NSAID
    b) anticoagulant
    d) fluoroquinolone

16. Medicare Part B covers inpatient or hospital type services.
    a) True
    b) False

17. Adverse drug events should be reported through the Med Watch program to which organization?
    a) DEA
    b) CMS
    c) FDA
    d) NABP

18. National Association of Boards of Pharmacy meets throughout the year to make and enforce laws.
    a) True
    b) False

19. Which of the following drugs is a calcium channel blocker used to treat hypertension?
    a) Zyloprim
    b) Cardizem CD
    c) Seroquel
    d) Eskalith

20. The pharmacy phone rings and it is Sally, a nurse with a local physician's office, wanting to call in a new prescription order. The pharmacist is busy counseling a patient at the window. As the technician answering the phone, you should…
    a) Take the order because the pharmacist on duty is too busy.
    b) Alert Sally that the pharmacist is busy and place her on hold until he is finished.
    c) Allow the senior technician to take the order because she has more experience.
    d) Put Sally on hold and forget about her….she forgot about you the last time you called her!

21. If a patient needed treatment for GERD, which of these drugs would most likely be prescribed?
    a) lithium carbonate
    b) alprazolam
    c) quetiapine
    d) omeprazole

22. Because of the Poison Prevention Act of 1970, we must place all medications in childproof containers regardless of patient preference.
    a) True
    b) False

23. A patient must have both Medicare Part A and Part B to enroll into _____ coverage.
    a) Part C
    b) Part D
    c) Both Part C and Part D
    d) Neither Part C nor Part D

24. Which of the following is a Class 4 (CIV) controlled substance indicated for anxiety disorder?'
    a) Eskalith
    b) Xanax
    c) Seroquel
    d) Vicodin

25. Which of these things are not within the scope of practice for a pharmacy technician.
    a) verifying another technician's work for dispensing meds to a patient
    b) typing information from the prescription into the computer database
    c) counting/pouring medications to be dispensed
    d) checking out patients at the cash register

26. A pharmacy technician at the cash register has asked a patient if they had any questions or would like to speak directly with the pharmacist about their medications. Which of the federal pharmacy laws is the technician abiding by?
    a) Health Insurance Portability and Accountability Act
    b) FDA Modernization Act
    c) Omnibus Budget Reconciliation Act
    d) Kefauver-Harris Amendment

27. Which of the following does JCAHO strive to improve through their accreditation requirements?
    a) patient safety
    b) performance improvement
    c) quality assurance
    d) all of these

28. A patient is sick with a terminal illness for which there is no known cure but a new drug being tested offers some hope of remission. The patient is able to use that medication through what Federal Law?
    a) Orphan Drug Act
    b) FDA Modernization Act
    c) Omnibus Budget Reconciliation Act
    d) Kefauver-Harris Amendment

29. It is unlawful for a technician to counsel a patient or perform other activities that require a pharmacist's professional judgment.
    a) True
    b) False

30. What government organization pays the Prescription Drug Plan premiums for Medicare Part D patients who are eligible by income limits and resources ?
    a) Food and Drug Administration
    b) Centers for Medicare and Medicaid Services
    c) Social Security Administration
    d) Drug Enforcement Administration

31. A patient presents at the pharmacy counter and requests to purchase a product that contains psuedoephedrine as one of its active ingredients. The clerk at the counter asks the customer for her picture ID and signature. The clerk and the patient are following what major law?
    a) FDA Modernization Act
    b) Controlled Substance Act
    c) Behind-The-Counter Act
    d) Combat Meth Act

32. A well diversely trained, knowledgeable and certified technician will be more marketable and desired.
    a) True
    b) False

33. Levofloxacin is indicated for various types of infection but which age group should not use this drug?
    a) less than 18 years
    b) 19 to 60 years
    c) over 60 years
    d) none of these

34. The Prescription Drug Marketing Act – A law requiring many medications for animals to be ordered by a veterinarian and have similar labeling as would the human medication counterparts – was passed in _____.
    a) 1970
    b) 1987
    c) 1990
    d) 1993

35. The Joint Commission group must announce to the facility the dates of their next scheduled inspection.
    a) True
    b) False

36. Which pair of medications listed are classed as antipsychotic agents?
    a) levofloxacin and amoxicillin
    b) lithium carbonate and quetiapine
    c) hydrocodone/acetaminophen and ibuprofen
    d) alprazolam and diltiazem

37. What organization is responsible for overseeing the pharmacies, the hospitals and other facilities where medications are used, as well as, those employed who are involved in the dispensing process (i.e. pharmacists, technicians, physicians, nurses etc…) in a particular state?
    a) NABP
    b) SBOP
    c) FDA
    d) DEA

38. The ratio laws only count the technicians included in the dispensing process. Other technicians on duty can be doing other duties unrelated to the dispensing function.
    a) True
    b) False

39. The Health Insurance Portability and Accountability Act is enforced by whom?
    a) FDA
    c) SBOP
    b) DEA
    d) CMS

40. The drug _____ may cause reduced effectiveness of contraceptives.
    a) amoxicillin
    c) alprazolam
    b) omeprazole
    d) warfarin

41. The Medicare program governed by each of the individual states has various programs to assist Aged, Blind, Disabled, Pregnant women and Children under 18.
    a) True
    b) False

42. Which of the following drug's actions can be reversed by using Vitamin K?
    a) Vicodin
    c) Xanax
    b) Coumadin
    d) Levaquin

43. Good Manufacturing Practices were initiated to ensure the safety and effectiveness of all marketable drugs. What major law included these provisions?
    a) Health Insurance Portability and Accountability Act
    b) Omnibus Budget Reconciliation Act
    c) FDA Modernization Act
    d) Kefauver-Harris Amendment

44. In the hospital or healthcare pharmacy setting, which of the following is not permissible for technicians?
    a) Filling an automated dispensing machine with floor stock
    b) Preparation of intravenous admixtures
    c) Monthly unit inspections for expired pharmaceuticals
    d) Receiving a verbal order from a physician or nurse
    e) Picking medications for the unit dose cart fill

45. The Pharmacist-In-Charge is responsible for overseeing all staff and the daily operations of a pharmacy.
    a) True
    b) False

46. Which of the medications listed carries a warning of increased risks of serious Cardiovascular events?
    a) diltiazem
    c) montelukast
    b) ibuprofen
    d) alprazolam

47. A pharmacy technician is preparing a medication for a pediatric patient that must be compounded because the medication does not come in a liquid form. Which law allows this process?
    a) Health Insurance Portability and Accountability Act
    b) FDA Modernization Act
    c) Omnibus Budget Reconciliation Act
    d) Kefauver-Harris Amendment

48. NABP's mission is to help assist its member boards to develop and implement uniform pharmacy standards.
    a) True   b) False

49. The Harrison Narcotic Act was the first attempt at preventing drug trafficking by requiring a prescription to obtain opium.
    a) True   b) False

50. Which of the following pairs of medications are indicated for pain?
    a) Seroquel and Eskalith   c) Lortab and Motrin
    b) Coumadin and Xanax   d) Levaquin and Xanax

51. The 1951 Durham-Humphrey Amendment made changes to previous laws. What did it require?
    a) A prescription for opium containing products
    b) The legend "Caution: Federal Law prohibits dispensing without a prescription" or the Rx only symbol.
    c) Childproof caps on all feasible containers
    d) Package inserts to be included with medications.

52. The FDA regulates both the practice of pharmacy and also sales and distribution of drugs on the market.
    a) True   b) False

53. Which of the following medications is indicated for treatment of asthma?
    a) montelukast   c) quetiapine
    b) alprazolam   d) omeprazole

54. A pharmacy technician should wear a nametag while on duty.
    a) True   b) False

55. Which of the following agencies handles the accreditation of healthcare organizations throughout the country through evaluations and inspections?
    a) FDA
    b) JCAHO
    c) NABP
    d) DEA

56. A technician can give a verbal copy to transfer a prescription to another pharmacy.
    a) True
    b) False

57. Even if it is not known for sure whether a medication or medical device caused an adverse event it should still be reported through the Med Watch Program.
    a) True
    b) False

58. Which of the following drugs is indicated for the treatment of pain and inflammation?
    a) montelukast
    b) allopurinol
    c) ibuprofen
    d) alprazolam

59. Personal Health Information cannot be repeated or released without proper authorization. This concept is known as _____.
    a) personality
    b) mortality
    c) liability
    d) confidentiality

60. Regardless of the training and experience a technician has, he/she must always work directly underneath the supervision of a licensed pharmacist.
    a) True
    b) False

61. The original 1906 Food and Drug Act was rewritten and passed into effect in 1938 to force "may be habit forming" warnings on all controlled substances and to bring regulations to what other substances?
    a) Alcohol
    b) Opium
    c) Cosmetics
    d) Animals

Match the following drugs to their generic names.

62.	Coumadin	_____	a) ibuprofen
63.	Singulair	_____	b) levofloxacin
64.	Zyloprim	_____	c) montelukast
65.	Levaquin	_____	d) lithium carbonate
66.	Lorcet	_____	e) amoxicilllin
67.	Eskalith	_____	f) quetiapine
68.	Motrin	_____	g) alprazolam
69.	Cardizem CD	_____	h) omeprazole
70.	Seroquel	_____	i) hydrocodone/acetaminophen
71.	Xanax	_____	j) warfarin
72.	Amoxil	_____	k)diltiazem CD
73.	Prilosec	_____	l) allopurinol

Match the following drugs to their classifications.

74.	Hydrocodone/Acetaminophen	_____	a) NSAID
75.	Levofloxacin	_____	b) anti-gout
76.	Ibuprofen	_____	c) anti-coagulant
77.	Montelukast	_____	d) proton pump inhibitor
78.	Allopurinol	_____	e) benzodiazepine
79.	Omeprazole	_____	f) calcium channel blocker
80.	Diltiazem CD	_____	g) leukotriene receptor antagonist
81.	Warfarin	_____	h) penicillin derivative antibiotic
82.	Amoxicillin	_____	i) opioid analgesic
83.	Alprazolam	_____	j)schizophrenic agent
84.	Quetiapine	_____	k)fluoroquinolone agent
85.	Lithium Carbonate	_____	l) manic-depressive agent

Round the following to the nearest tenth

86. 0.76

87. 0.23

Round the following to the nearest hundredth

88. 13.186

89. 101.289

Round the following to the nearest thousandth.

90. 2.08653

91. 487.0521

92. 36.8994

Change the following decimals to percent form.

93. 0.28

94. 0.015

95. 0.92

96. 0.418

Change the following percents to decimal form.

97. 49.5%

98. 32.1%

99. 0.025%

100. 4.15%

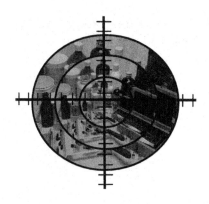

Mission 2:
Code words, Conversions
and Abbreviations

Mission Objectives:

*To become familiar with general medical terminology, prefixes and suffixes.

*To interpret sig codes and routes of administration in order to read prescriptions.

*To learn many of the abbreviations and acronyms used in pharmacy practice.

*To learn the chemical symbols and formulas commonly used in pharmacy.

*To recognize those abbreviations known to be error prone that should be avoided)

*To become familiar with the systems of measurement used in pharmacy practice.

*To master the conversions between the various units of measurement.

* To master the rules of using Roman Numerals

*To gain baseline knowledge of twelve of the most popular drugs on the market.

*To brush up on basic mathematical skills of fractions, ratios, decimals and percents.

There are many **abbreviations** that will be used in pharmacy practice. Working in an institutional pharmacy, a technician will read and input data from physician's orders on a daily basis. In the ambulatory care setting, a technician will also interpret prescriptions that are written by physicians. A technician should be familiar with these because they are used so regularly. Even though certain abbreviations and/or codes are recognized to be easily misinterpreted and are recommended by organizations to be avoided, many practitioners will continue to use them. Therefore it is important for us to be knowledgeable of all common pharmacy terminology.

Some are abbreviations or **symbols** for certain terms. Others are either **root words, prefixes or suffixes**, that when placed together mean a specific term. For instance, Osteoporosis-Osteo meaning bone, por(e) meaning hole, osis meaning condition. Therefore, one could assume that the term Osteoporosis is a condition where there are holes in the bone.

Also included in this chapter are abbreviations for the **routes of administration** and **sig codes**. Most of these type abbreviations are derived from Latin terms and if known, the Latin terminology will be included. Last and final there is a list of **common conversions** that will be necessary to learn in order to perform basic pharmaceutical calculations. The conversion of weights and measures can be confusing at times because there are several different systems still in use with today's society.

The **metric system,** adopted in 1960, was created to standardize measurement around the world) Most pharmacies prefer to use this system because it is so easy to use. Every unit of measure is based on the number ten so calculations are much easier to perform.

Even though the metric system is the standard, many times conversions will have to be carried out in order to correctly dispense or compound the right amount of medication. Many practitioners, especially the older physicians, still use the systems that were in place and common in the early years of their medical practice.

The **avoirdupois system**, for instance, is still used quite often. It is a system of weight. Another system used primarily to measure liquid is known as the **apothecary system.** Still yet another system that patients will be most familiar with is the **household system.** Usually when a medication is dispensed, the dosage is converted over to the household system so it's more easily understood by the common patient to ensure the correct dosage is given.

Miscellaneous Abbreviations and Acronyms

In the medical arena there are so many acronyms and abbreviations that we use. These listed below are those used more commonly and some that you may be asked to interpret on a daily basis. You might find some of these listed on medication orders or prescriptions regularly received in the pharmacy.

ADE – Adverse Drug Event
Amp- ampule
AWP – average wholesale price
BP – blood pressure
CBC – Complete blood count
C/S -Culture and sensitivity
DOB – date of birth
EKG – electrocardiogram
Hx – History
I/O – intake and output
OJ – orange juice
PDP – Prescription Drug Plan
post-partum – after delivery
R- Respirations
Rx - recipe or prescription
T – temperature
TPN – total parental nutrition
VO – verbal order

ADS – Automated Dispensing System
ASAP – as soon as possible
BM – bowel movement
BS – blood sugar
CCU – coronary/critical care unit
D/C – discontinue or discharge
Dx – diagnosis
HMO – Health Maintenance Organization
ICU – intensive care unit
MI- myocardial infarction (heart attack)
OTC – over the counter
post-op – after surgery
pre-op – before surgery
RBC – red blood cells
STAT – now, immediately
TO – telephoned order
USP – US Pharmacopoeia
WBC – white blood cells

Abbreviations of Illnesses and Disease States

Oftentimes you will see these abbreviations of common disease states and illnesses as an inclusion on your prescriptions or medication orders. If a prescriber has listed a "condition" for which a patient is taking a medication, then you would want to include it in with the directions. However, just because we often know the primary indication for many medications, unless a prescriber specifies or the patient requests it, we generally do not include it with the labeled directions.

ADD – Attention Deficit Disorder	ADHD – Attention Deficit Hyperactivity Disorder
AIDS –Acquired immunodeficiency syndrome	BPH - Benign prostatic hypertrophy
CAD – Coronary Artery Disease	CF – Cystic Fibrosis
CHF – Congestive heart failure	COPD– Chronic Obstructive Pulmonary Disease
CRF- Chronic Renal Failure	DM – Diabetes Mellitus
ESRD – End Stage Renal Disease	GAD- Generalized Anxiety Disorder
GERD – gastro esophageal reflux disease	H/A - Headache
HBP – High Blood Pressure	HIV – human immunodeficiency virus
HTN – Hypertension	HPV – Human Papilloma Virus
IBS – Irritable Bowel Syndrome	INR - International normalizing ratio
MI- myocardial infarction (heart attack)	MRSA- Methicillin-resistant Staphylococcus aureus
N/V –nausea and vomiting	OCD – Obsessive Compulsive Disorder
OM- Otitis Media (middle ear infection)	PMS – Premenstrual Syndrome
PUD –peptic ulcer disease	RA – Rheumatoid Arthritis
SOB – Shortness of Breath	TB – tuberculosis
URI – upper respiratory infection	UTI – urinary tract infection

Common Chemical Symbols and Formulas

We use many chemical symbols and formulas on a day to day basis. These are the more common ones. If you have previously studied Chemistry then you are probably more familiar with these than anyone who has not been exposed to that type of information. The subscripted or superscripted numbers (those below and above the normal print line) are part of the formulas. Though you need not understand that those numbers have to do with the makeup of the molecules listed, you would want to "memorize" the numbers as part of the formula name. For instance, the water formula below would be referred to as "H two O".

Symbols

C – Carbon
Ca – Calcium
Cl – Chlorine
Fe – Iron
H – Hydrogen
I – Iodine

K – Potassium
Mg – Magnesium
Na – Sodium
O – Oxygen
S – Sulfur
Zn – Zinc

Formulas

$AgNO_3$ – Silver Nitrate
$CaCO_3$ – Calcium Carbonate
CO_2 – Carbon Dioxide
$FeSO_4$ – Ferrous Sulfate
HCl – Hydrochloride
H_2O_2 – Hydrogen Peroxide

H_2O – Water
KCl – Potassium Chloride
MgO – Magnesium Oxide
**$MgSO_4$ – Magnesium Sulfate
NaCl – Sodium Chloride
$NaHCO_3$ – Sodium Bicarbonate
O_2 – Oxygen
ZnO – Zinc Oxide

Being able to recognize part of a word can help you determine what that word is. The following lists of prefixes and suffixes are ones used in our day to day pharmacy and medical practices. These before (prefixes) and after (suffixes) parts of words can drastically change their meanings.

General Medical Prefixes

anti – inhibiting
brady – slow
endo – inside
hypo – low
macro – large
neo – new
poly – many
sub – below

ante – before
contra – against
gluc- sugar
inter – between
mal – abnormal
patho – disease
post – after
tachy – fast

auto – self regulating
dys – pain
hyper – high/excessive
intra – within
micro – very small
peri – around
pre – before

Medical Prefixes for areas of the body

arterio – artery
derm – skin
hepato – liver
opth- eye
phlebo – vein
psych – mental, mind

cardio – heart
gastro – stomach
myo – muscle
osteo – bone
pneumo, pulmo – lung
rhine – nasal

colo – colon
hemo – blood
nephro – kidney
oto – ear
procto – anal, rectal
vaso – blood vessels

Medical Prefixes for colors

chlor – green   cirrh – yellow   cyan – blue
erythr – red   melan – black   leuk – white

Medical Suffixes

algia – pain   ary – pertaining to
asthenia – weakness   cide, cidal – killing
cyst – bladder   cyte- cell
derm – skin   ectomy – removal
gram – record   iasis – condition
itis – inflammation   ology – study of
meter – measuring instrument   oma – tumor
opia – vision   osis – abnormal condition
pathy – disease   penia – decrease
phage – of or pertaining to eating/ingestion   rrhea – discharge
sclerosis – narrowing, constriction   scope – examining instrument
spasm – involuntary contraction   stasis – stop or stand

Routes of Administration

To define the word "route" we could simply say, a pathway from one place to another. Therefore as we define the phrase, "Route of Administration" we are referring to the pathway that medications get into the body. These will be some of the building blocks that make up the directions for use that practitioners will use when writing orders or prescriptions. It is very important that these abbreviations and their meanings are planted firmly in your memory. These will be the foundation of your daily activities in the pharmacy profession.

ad – right ear   *auris dexter*   as – left ear   *auris sinister*
au – both/each ear *auris utro*   buc – buccal or inside cheek
IM – intramuscular   inj – injection *injectio*
IV – intravenous   IVPB – intravenous piggyback
npo – nothing by mouth *non per os*   od – right eye *oculus dexter*
os – left eye   *oculus sinister*   ou – both/each eye *oculus utro*
po – by mouth   *per os*   PR – per rectum or rectally
sl – sublingual or under tongue   sq – subcutaneous
TD – transdermally   vag – vaginally

JCAHO has released an official "do not use" (DNU) list of abbreviations for the organizations they accredit. Because these abbreviations are still used in some settings you will still need to learn them. Abbreviations notated with ** are included on this do not use list. Those notated with * are suggested to be avoided and may be included in a future DNU list. A similar and more inclusive list has been endorsed by the Institute for Safe Medicine Practices.

33

Dosage Forms

Medications can be available in many different dosage forms based on the needs of the patient. These are some of the more common examples.

AQ – water   *aqua*
cr - cream
inh - inhalant
liq – liquid *liquor*
MDI – metered dose inhaler
ung – ointment *ungentum*
tab – tablet *tabella*

Cap – capsule *capsula*
elix – elixir *liquor*
inj – injection *injectico*
lot - lotion
syr – syrup   *syrupus*
supp – suppository *suppositorium*

Dosage Release Form Accronyms

Medications come in different release forms. Most often, all of the active ingredient will be released at once when it is dissolved in the gut. However, some medications have been altered so that they will release over a period of hours or days. The latter has several different versions.

CR – controlled release
DR – delayed release
DS – double strength
EC – enteric coated
ER – extended release

HS – half strength
IR – immediate release
LA – long acting
XR – extended release

Recon Mission 2:

There are currently two major organizations that have recommendations/guidelines for dangerous abbreviations. You should visit both of these sites and print copies of both lists of recommended abbreviations to avoid) Study both lists and familiarize yourself with those abbreviations.

- **The Joint Commission** implemented the official "Do Not Use List". Go to their website at www.jcaho.org then choose "Topics" then "Patient Safety" then choose "The Official Do Not Use List".

- **The Institute for Safe Medication Practices** has a list of "Error-Prone abbreviations". Go to their website at www.ismp.org then choose "Medication Safety Tools and Resources" then choose "Error-Prone Abbreviations"

Sig Codes

The phrase "sig code" is translated from the Latin word "Signa" which means "to write". Therefore our sig codes are an abbreviation of what the prescriber wants to write. These are also very important to commit to your memory as you will be using these throughout your entire pharmacy technician career. Note that some are included on the Joint Commission's Do Not Use list or are suggested to be avoided) You still want to be familiar with all of these abbreviations.

a – before *ante*	ac – before meals *ante cibum*
ad lib – as desired	am – in the morning *ante meridian*
bid – twice daily *bis in die*	c – with *cum*
et – and *et*	gtt – drop *guttae*
h – hour *hora*	hs – at bedtime *hora somni*
nr – no refill	p – after *post*
pc – after meals *post cibum*	per – by or through
pm – in the evening *post meridian*	prn – as needed *pro re nata*
q – each, every *quaque*	q#h – every # hours *quaque # hora*
q46h – every 4 to 6 hours	**qd - daily *quaque die*
qid – four times daily *quater in die*	**qod – every other day
qs – quantity sufficient *quantum sufficiat*	s – without *sine*
ss – one half	stat – now, immediately *statim*
tid – three times daily *ter in die*	ud, ut dict – as directed *ut dictum*
x – times	

Measurement Abbreviations

*cc – cubic centimeter
gal – gallon
kg – kilogram
mcg – microgram *μg
mL or mL – milliliter
qt – quart

cm – centimeter
gr – grain
L – Liter
mEq – milliequivalent
oz – ounce
Tbsp – tablespoon

g – gram
**I.U. – international units
lb – pound
mg – milligram
pt – pint
tsp – teaspoon

These Apothecary symbols are sometimes still used today even though their use is highly discouraged.

ℨ Dram   ℥ Fluid Ounce

Conversion Equivalents

When you are performing pharmaceutical calculations, unless otherwise specified, ALWAYS use the metric values. They make your calculations much easier.

Conversions must often be performed before, during or after a pharmaceutical calculation. Oftentimes, conversions will need to be performed between the major measurement systems and other times the conversions will be between larger and smaller units within the same measurement system.

Metric Equivalents

1000 micro liters = 1milliliter
1000 micrograms = 1 milligram
1000 grams   = 1 kilogram

1000milliliters   = 1 liter
1000milligrams = 1 gram
1 kilogram = 2.2 pounds

Volume Measurement Conversions

Metric	Apothecary	Household
1mL		15 gtts
5mL	1 dram	1 tsp
10mL	2 drams	2 tsp
15mL	½ fl oz	1 Tbsp
30mL	1 fl oz	2 Tbsp
60mL	2 fl oz	¼ cup
120mL	4 fl oz	½ cup
180mL	6 fl oz	¾ cup
240mL	8 fl oz	1 cup
480mL	16fl oz or 473mL	1 pint
960mL	32fl oz or 946mL	1 quart
3840mL	128oz fl	1 gallon

Weight Measurement Conversions

Metric	Apothecary	Household	Avoirdupois
0.4mg	gr 1/150		
15mg	gr ¼		
30mg	gr ½		
60 or 65mg	gr 1		gr 1
325mg	gr 5		
650mg	gr 10		
30g		1 oz	28.35g
60g		2 oz	
120g		4 oz	
240g		8 oz	
480g		16 oz or 1lb	454g
1 kg		2.2lbs	

The abbreviation for grains (gr) is typically written in front of the numerical amount.
The correct abbreviation for gram is g but you are likely to see it written gm from time to time.

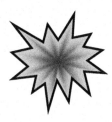

Math Blaster

Continue with some very basic math skills. The lessons learned in this mission are the very building blocks of much more complicated pharmacy calculations. Let the rules and practice take root and grow for in the future missions they will be used many times over again.

Roman Numerals

Roman Numerals were used long ago to represent a numerical system. The system was based on letters representing numbers. By using only seven letters, any number could be notated)

Letter	Value
I	1
V	5
X	10
L	50
C	100
D	500
M	1000

It may seem strange that we would still be using this system today but many practitioners like Roman Numerals because they are much harder to defraud or alter on prescriptions. There are only a few rules for working with Roman Numerals and the best way to learn them is to just jump right in.

Using these principle rules below, note the examples which are correct and incorrect.

* A letter cannot be repeated more than three times in a row.
  III is correct   XXXX is incorrect
* Consecutive letters of the same value are added together.
  II equals a value of 2 (1 + 1 = 2)
* Do not repeat letters that can be represented by another letter.
  XX is a correct value of 20
  VV is incorrect because 5 + 5 = 10 which is represented by X
* If a letter is followed by one of lesser value they are added together.
  VII equals a value of 7 (5 + 1 + 1 = 7)
* If a letter is followed by one of greater value then the previous value is subtracted from the latter value.
  IX equals a value of 9 (1 subtracted from 10 or 10 – 1 = 9)
* Only one number may be subtracted from another.
  IV is a correct value of 4 (1 subtracted from 5 or 5 – 1 = 9)
  IIV is incorrect because two numbers cannot be subtracted.
* Only powers of ten may be subtracted. (1, 10, 100)
  XC is a correct value of 90 (10 subtracted from 100 or 100 – 10 = 90)
  VC is incorrect because a value of 5 cannot be subtracted.

Fractions, Ratios, Decimals and Percents

With pharmacy calculations, oftentimes it is necessary to convert between fractions, ratios, decimals and percents. In mission 1, decimals and percents were introduced) Here, the fractions and ratios will be brought in. You should be familiar with all of these numerical forms and how to change between them. Whatever type of calculation is being performed determines what form of number is needed) For instance, you may be calculating a compounding problem and need a percent form to go in your formula but you have only been given a ratio to work with. There must be a conversion from ratio to percent in order for you to work the problem.

Ratio to Fraction or Fraction to Ratio Conversion

When changing from ratio to fraction the task is simple. A ratio is listed with two numbers separated by a colon (:) The number listed first becomes the numerator or top number of the fraction. The number listed second becomes the denominator or the bottom number of the fraction. To reverse the process, the numerator of the fraction becomes the first part of the ratio. Add a colon and then the denominator of the fraction as the second number.

1:3 $\longrightarrow$	$\dfrac{1}{3}$	$\dfrac{3}{4}$ $\longrightarrow$	becomes 3:4
becomes			

If necessary, the fraction or ratio can be simplified or reduced to lowest terms. To do this, divide the numerator and denominator fraction numbers (or the first and second ratio numbers by the same number.)

$\underline{2}$ (both numbers can be divided equally by 2) $2 \div 2 = \underline{1}$

4 $4 \div 2 = 2$

Therefore $\underline{2}$ reduces to $\underline{1}$

4 $\longrightarrow$ 2

5:100 (both numbers can be divided equally by 5)

$5 \div 5 = 1$ $100 \div 5 = 20$

Therefore 5 : 100 reduces to 1 : 20

Fraction to Decimal or Decimal to Fraction Conversion

Converting fractions to decimals and vice versa can be a little more tricky but no more difficult than earlier lessons. The line in a fraction means "to divide" so converting fractions to decimals involves a mere step in division.

$\underline{5}$
8   actually could be translated into $5 \div 8$

Therefore $\underline{5}$ becomes 0.625 in decimal form.
8

Doing the opposite, going from decimal to fraction requires a little more effort.

0.125 is a decimal number form. The denominator is determined by the place value of the digit on the far right. The number "5" is in the thousandths place. That means that the number "1000" would become the denominator of this fraction. Once that takes place the leading zero and the decimal point could be discarded)

0.125 becomes $\underline{125}$
      $\longrightarrow$ 1000   this fraction can now be reduced

$\underline{125}$ Both numerator and denominator can be equally divided by 125
1000 $125 \div 125 = 1$ $1000 \div 125 = 8$

$\underline{125}$ becomes $\underline{1}$
1000 $\longrightarrow$ 8

Decimal to Percent and Percent to Decimal Conversion

This process was introduced in Mission 1 so if need be, revisit that former lesson and brush up. As a reminder here, when going from decimal to percent form simply move the decimal two places to the right and add the percent sign. (%) When going from percent to decimal, drop the % sign and change to a decimal, then move that decimal two places to the left. Here are the illustrations to help you remember.

.D P $\longrightarrow$ D P . $\longrightarrow$ %

.D P $\longleftarrow$ D P . $\longleftarrow$ %

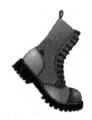

Drill Practice

Complete the following and then check yourself in the rear of the textbook.

Determine the value of the Roman Numerals given:

5. XXX
6. XII
7. IX
8. XC

9. LX
10. XIV
11. M
12. XLII

Write the numbers in Roman Numeral form:

13. 20
14. 28
15. 40
16. 10

17. 7
18. 15
19. 16
20. 8

Fill in the following chart with the appropriate value.

Ratio	Fraction	Decimal	Percent
3:4			
	$\frac{3}{5}$		
		0.63	
2:3			
			42%
7:8			
			36%
	$\frac{1}{8}$		
		0.04	
1:4			

Drug Training Chapter Two

Brand Name	Generic Name	Drug Classification	Primary Indication	Side effects, Warnings, Other
Glucovance	Glyburide/ Metformin	Anti-Diabetic Combination (Sulfonylurea/ Biguanide)	Type 2 Diabetes	Upper respiratory infection, headache, GI upset, dizziness
Lodine	Etodolac	NSAID Non-Steroidal Anti-Inflammatory	Osteoarthritis, Rheumatoid Arthritins and for acute pain	May increase risk of serious cardiovascular thrombotic events, myocardial infarction, and stroke; may also cause gastrointestinal disturbances abnormal renal function, anemia, dizziness, edema, elevated liver enzymes, headaches, increased bleeding time, pruritis, rashes, tinnitus
Zoloft	Sertraline	Selective Serotonin Reuptake Inhibitor	Major Depressive Disorder in adults	May increase risk of suicidal thinking and behavior in children, adolescents, and young adults Headache, Dizziness, Somnolence, Insomnia, Dry Mouth, Diarrhea,
Hytrin	Terazosin	Alpha-1 adrenoceptor blocker	Symptomatic benign prostatic hyperplasia or hypertension	Asthenia, postural hypotension, dizziness, somnolence, nasal congestion/rhinitis, and impotence
Zetia	Ezetimibe	Lipid-lowering Agent	Alone or in Adjunctive Hyperlipidemia therapy	May increase risk of Rhabdomyolysis and myopathy and/or cause abnormal liver enzyme levels, upper respiratory tract infection, diarrhea, arthralgia, sinusitis, and pain in extremities
Ambien, Ambien CR	Zolpidem	C IV Hypnotic	Insomnia	Daytime drowsiness, Dizziness, Headache, Nausea & Vomiting

Brand Name	Generic Name	Drug Classification	Primary Indication	Side effects, Warnings, Other
Klor-Con	Potassium Chloride	Potassium Supplement	Hypokalemia (low blood potassium)	Hyperkalemia, nausea, vomiting, flatulence, abdominal pain/discomfort and diarrhea
Lexapro	Escitalopram	Selective Serotonin Reuptake Inhibitor	Depression, Major Depressive Disorder, Generalized Anxiety Disorder	May increase risk of suicidal thinking and behavior in children, adolescents, and young adults, may cause nausea, ejaculation disorder, fatigue, insomnia
Cozaar	Losartan	Angiotensin II receptor blocker (ARB)	Hypertension	Should be avoided during pregnancy; may cause upper respiratory infection, cough, dizziness, diarrhea, insomnia
Toprol XL	Metoprolol Extended Release	Beta-adrenergic recepter blocker	Hypertension, Angina Pectoris	tiredness, dizziness, depression, diarrhea, shortness of breath, bradycardia, and rash
Tylox, Percocet	Oxycodone/ Acetaminophen	C II Opioid Analgesic	Moderate to Moderately Severe Pain	Light-headedness, Dizziness, Drowsiness, Nausea & Vomiting
Prozac	Fluoxetine	Selective Serotonin Reuptake Inhibitor	Major Depressive Disorder, Obsessive Compulsive Disorder, Bulimia Nervosa and Panic Disorder	May increase risk of suicidal thinking and behavior in children, adolescents, and young adults, may cause nausea, decreased libido, fatigue, insomnia, Should not be used in combination with an MAOI

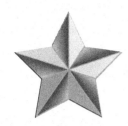

Mission 2 Debriefing

Answer the following questions in assessment of the lessons learned in Mission 2. For best results, repeat the exercise until no questions are missed then move on to the next mission.

Fill in the missing information on the following.

1. _____ –acquired immunodeficiency syndrome
2. N/V - _____
3. D/C – _____
4. _____ – as soon as possible
5. DOB – _____
6. Dx - _____
7. _____ – enteric coated
8. _____ – intake and output
9. pre-op – _____
10. LA – _____
11. _____ – congestive heart failure
12. _____ – now, immediately
13. _____ – total parental nutrition
14. USP – _____
15. XR – _____

16. _____ – History
17. _____ – urinary tract infection
18. _____ – gastro esophageal reflux disease
19. BP – _____
20. AWP – _____
21. _____ - over the counter
22. BS - _____
23. _____ - intensive care unit
24. _____ - after surgery
25. post-partum - _____
26. VO - _____
27. _____ -human immunodeficiency virus
28. _____ -   electrocardiogram
29. BM - _____
30. PDP - _____

Write the correct symbol or formula for the following.

31. _____ - Potassium
32. _____ - Magnesium
33. _____ - Calcium
34. _____ - Iron
35. _____ - Water
36. _____ - Sodium
37. _____ - Zinc

38. _____ - Ferrous Sulfate
39. _____ - Silver Nitrate
40. _____ - Potassium Chloride
41. _____ - Calcium Carbonate
42. _____ - Hydrogen Peroxide
43. _____ - Sodium Bicarbonate
44. _____ - Sodium Chloride

Fill in the body areas to which these prefixes pertain.

45. nephro- _____   53. arterio- _____
46. pulmo- _____   54. cardio- _____
47. rhine- _____   55. colo-_____
48. vaso- _____   56. gastro-_____
49. hepato-_____   57. pneumo - _____
50. myo- _____   58. derm - _____
51. osteo-_____   59. phlebo - _____
52. procto-_____   60. oto - _____

What prefixes represent the colors listed below?

61. blue -_____   64. green -_____
62. yellow -_____   65. black -_____
63. red - _____   66. whitc - _____

Match the following suffixes to their meanings.

67. itis   _____a) eating/ingestion
68. pathy   _____b) study of
69. ectomy   _____c) inflammation
70. ology   _____d) condition
71. iasis   _____e. tumor
72. spasm   _____f. disease
73. phage   _____g. removal of
74. oma   _____h. involuntary contraction

List the abbreviations of these routes of administration.

75. _____ - left ear   80. _____ - vaginally   85. _____ - left eye
76. _____ - by mouth   81. _____ - intraveneous   86. _____ - transdermally
77. _____ - intramuscular   82. _____ - right ear   87. _____ - each ear
78. _____ - both eyes   83. _____ - rectally   88. _____ - buccal
79. _____ - sublingual   84. _____ - subcutaneous   89. _____ - right eye

Choose the best sig code for the expanded directions for use .

90. Take two tablets now, then one tablet every four hours as needed.
    a) 2 tabs stat, then 1 tab q46h prn
    b) 2 tabs stat, then 1 tab q4h prn
    c) 2 tabs then 1 tab prn
    d) 2 tabs stat, then q4h prn

91. Unwrap and insert one suppository rectally at bedtime as needed.
    a) 1supp hs prn
    b) 1 supp pr prn
    c) 1 supp pr hs prn
    d) 1 supp pr hs

92. Take two tablespoonfuls by mouth before meals and at bedtime.
    a) 2 Tbsp achs
    b) 2 Tbsp po achs
    c) 2 tsp po achs
    d) 2 Tbsp po pchs

93. Instill three drops in left ear four times daily.
    a) iii gtts os qid
    b) iii gtts ad qid
    c) iii gtts as qid
    d) iii gtts au qid

94. Take two tablespoonfuls by mouth after meals and at bedtime.
    a) 2 Tbsp achs
    b) 2 Tbsp po achs
    c) 2 tsp po achs
    d) 2 Tbsp po pchs

95. Take two tablespoonfuls by mouth three times daily as needed.
    a) 2 tsp tid prn
    b) 2 tsp po tid prn
    c) 2 Tbsp po tid prn
    d) 2 tsp po tid

96. Take one tablet by mouth every other day as directed.
    a) 1 tab po qd ud
    b) 1 tab po qd
    c) 1 tab po qod ud
    d) 1 tab po ud

97. Take one teaspoonful by mouth twice daily.
    a) 1tsp po bid prn
    b) 1tsp bid
    c) 1tsp po tid
    d) 1tsp po bid

98. Inject subcutaneously 25 units every morning and 10 units every evening.
    a) 25units sq qam et 15units qpm
    b) 25units sq qam et 10units qpm
    c) 25units i.v. qam et 10units qpm
    d) none of these

99. Take two tablets by mouth every four to six hours.
    a) 2 tabs q46h prn
    b) 2 tabs po q46h prn
    c) 2 tabs po q46h
    d) none of these

100. Which of the following pairs of medications are indicated for Major Depressive Disorder?
    a) etolodac and sertraline
    b) escitalopram and fluoxetine
    c) losartan and metoprolol
    d) sertraline and losartan

101. The drug Zetia is indicated for _____.
    a) hyperlipidemia
    b) insomnia
    e) diabetes
    c) rheumatoid arthritis
    d) type 2

102. Which of the drugs below is indicated for BPH or benign prostatic hyperplasia?
    a) Cozaar
    b) Lodine
    c) Hytrin
    d) Toprol XL

103. According to DEA regulations, Ambien is known as a _____ controlled substance.
    a) C II
    b) C III
    c) C IV
    d) C V

104. Selective Serotonin Reuptake Inhibitors are used in treating depression and include all but which of the following medications?
    a) ezetimibe
    b) sertraline
    c) escitalopram
    d) fluoxetine

105. Lodine is a drug that warns an increased risk of _____.
    a) suicidal thinking and behavior in children, adolescents and young adults.
    b) rhabdomyolysis and myopathy.
    c) cardiovascular events such as blood clots, heart attacks and strokes.
    d) None of these

106. Terazosin, Losartan and Metoprolol are from different drug classifications but share a common indication of _____.
    a) insomnia
    b) pain
    c) diabetes
    d) hypertension

107. Which of the following pairs of medications are used in pain treatment?
    a) etodolac and oxycodone/acetaminophen
    b) Zoloft and Zetia
    c) etodolac and ezetimibe
    d) Tylox and Toprol XL

108. Which of these drugs cannot be written with refills?
    a) Ambien CR
    b) Lexapro
    c) Prozac
    d) Percocet

109. The drug Klor-Con is used to treat _____.
    a) insomnia
    b) hypokalemia
    c) osteoarthritis
    d) angina pectoris

Match the following drugs to their generic names.

110.	Ambien	_____ a)	fluoxetine
111.	Hytrin	_____ b)	oxycodone/acetaminophen
112.	Lodine	_____ c)	metoprol
113.	Prozac	_____ d)	losartan
114.	Toprol XL	_____ e)	escitalopram
115.	Lexapro	_____ f)	potassium chloride
116.	Zetia	_____ g)	zolpidem
117.	Zoloft	_____ h)	ezetimibe
118.	Glucovance	_____ i)	terazosin
119.	Tylox	_____ j)	sertraline
120.	Cozaar	_____ k)	etodolac
121.	Klor-Con	_____ l)	glyburide/metformin

Match the following drugs to their classifications.

122.	Oxycodone/Acetaminophen	_____ a)	anti-diabetic combination
123.	Losartan	_____ b)	NSAID
124.	Potassium Chloride	_____ c)	SSRI
125.	Ezetimibe	_____ d)	alpha-1 blocker
126.	Sertraline	_____ e)	lipid lowering agent
127.	Glyburide/Metformin	_____ f)	hypnotic
128.	Fluoxetine	_____ g)	potassium supplement
129.	Metoprolol extended release	_____ h)	SSRI
130.	Escitalopram	_____ i)	ARB
131.	Zolpidem	_____ j)	beta blocker
132.	Terazosin	_____ k)	opioid analgesic
133.	Etodolac	_____ l)	SSRI

Determine the value of the Roman Numerals given:

134.	XX		138.	LIV
135.	XI		139.	XV
136.	IV		140.	C
137.	CX		141.	XLIV

Write the numbers in Roman Numeral form:

142.	30		146.	9
143.	24		147.	17
144.	50		148.	6
145.	13		149.	4

Fill in the following chart with the appropriate value.

	Ratio	Fraction	Decimal	Percent
150.	1:3			
151.		2		
152.			0.46	
153.	5:8			
154.				50%
155.	2:3			

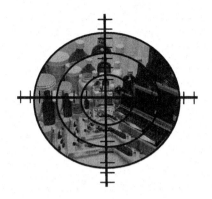

Mission 3:
Operation
Ambulatory Care

Mission Objectives

*To recognize the different types of pharmacies in ambulatory care.

*To become familiar with all aspects of the prescription filling process.

*To understand the various requirements for written, oral and electronic
  prescriptions and their dispensing labels.

*To become familiar with the equipment used in ambulatory practice.

*To become familiar with customer service principles and communication
  techniques.

*To gain baseline knowledge of twelve of the most popular drugs on the market.

*To understand the principles of pharmaceutical calculations used in the
  ambulatory setting including ratio and proportion dosage calculations, figuring
  days supply amounts, figuring insulin quantities and total quantities to be
  dispensed and DEA number validation.

Community, outpatient, ambulatory care pharmacies serve non-institutional "walk-in" patients. These pharmacies are found in a variety of settings. Chain (corporate) pharmacies, department or grocery store pharmacies, independent retail pharmacies, outpatient government facilities, and mail-order pharmacies all fit into this "ambulatory care" category.

Although prescription drug dispensing to ambulatory patients has increased tremendously in recent years, the increase has not been equally divided among all types of outpatient settings. Grocery store and chain pharmacies have grown significantly in number and volume of patients they serve. This has much to do with marketing and pricing strategies. Because these big box stores or their chain store competition do group purchasing, they are able to get contracts based on the amount of dollars spent nationally, all stores included.

Independent retail stores, on the other hand, are on the decline. The expenses of running a business are increasing each year, while reimbursement for medications and profit margin get lower each year. Unless an independent pharmacy has an excellent location and a large patient volume it can be tough to stay in business. Without the volume of purchasing, an independent store will likely have much higher contract pricing with the wholesalers and that could making remaining competitive locally difficult.

Other ambulatory care pharmacies would be found in government facilities such as military installations, VA hospitals and Indian Health Service facilities. These types of pharmacies sometimes have an advantage over retail stores, in that they normally do not handle the billing process. This would be handled in another department; usually a separate "billing office" takes care of this service. This is possible because patients who are eligible to use these services typically do not have an "out of pocket" cost at the time of receiving their medications. If they are responsible for their medication costs, it is likely done by sending out a monthly statement.

Mail-order pharmacies associated with an insurance coverage also have an advantage. Employees in this type of pharmacy do not have to meet the public eye-to-eye, though they will be working via telephone with them. We all know at times, this would definitely be to our advantage. Many corporate employers are going to this type of prescription drug service for their employees. It is less expensive in some cases for employers. Some patients may feel that their choice of pharmacies is being taken away because they are driven to use these mail order services because of cost savings.

For instance, a patient receiving a chronic blood pressure medication for a typical prescription of one pill daily with five refills may have to pay a $15.00 copayment at his local pharmacy. However, that same patient may be able to obtain a three months supply of that same chronic medication for the same copayment of $15.00. Therefore, patients are driven by the value of the dollar to use the mail order service. With all that being said, using a mail order service has some great advantages. Not only does a patient usually get better pricing, they also have the medications delivered discreetly right to their door/mailbox. For some patients, this is the best advantage of all.

The employees of the mail order pharmacy have the same responsibility to be courteous and friendly as those in "brick and mortar" pharmacies. Good customer service is what keeps patients coming back to the pharmacy month after month.

Similar to the mail order pharmacies that are associated with group or private prescription insurance coverage, Internet pharmacies are increasing due to the convenience opportunity. Patients using an Internet pharmacy can submit prescriptions to be filled several different ways. They can mail them in; have the prescriber call or fax them in directly to the Internet Pharmacy, have the Internet pharmacy call the prescriber's office to retrieve the prescription information or have the prescription transferred from another pharmacy.

The down side of using both mail order and Internet pharmacies is the time involved in receiving the medications. It would likely be an inconvenience if a patient needed something like an antibiotic for an infection right away but could be very simple for those repeat prescriptions for chronic medications.

Prescription or Non-Prescription

Medications are divided into two major categories: Prescription and Non-Prescription. Some non-Prescription medications can be bought over-the-counter without a prescription, thus we have the commonly used acronym OTC for those types of medications. These OTC medications have been approved by the FDA for patients who would like use a self-diagnosis and treatment option. These medications have been through stringent testing requirements and are labeled with specific instructions for safe use by the consumer.

Some non-Prescription medications require more information or restrictions on purchasing. These medications are commonly referred to as Behind-the-Counter or BTC medications. They can still be purchased without a prescription or medication order from the physician, however, their purchase is usually tracked by maintaining records. A patient or consumer would usually be required to show valid picture identification and often give demographic information such as name, address and date of birth in order to purchase.

Since most states require a consumer to be at least 18 years of age before purchasing any medication, age may also be a deciding factor in a BTC purchase. Other restrictions may also be in place due to the fact that a pharmacy, employer or even a state can have its own individual rules and policies. Note that some "Scheduled V or CV" cough syrups that contain a minimal amount of codeine may be available for purchase in this "BTC" class of medications. Though they are controlled substances, their abuse potential is generally very low and therefore, in some states this is allowed. Again note that this may not be permissible due to a state law prohibiting such or even a pharmacy's decision to avoid such sales of CV medications.

Prescription medications require a doctor's written or verbal order to be valid to be dispensed to a patient. Prescription medications are often referred to as "legend" drugs, due to the Federal law requirement (**1951- Durham-Humphrey Amendment)** that all prescription medication packaging displays the legend: Caution: Federal Law prohibits dispensing without a prescription.

In the first mission, the Controlled Substance Act of 1970 was reviewed. It indicated that medications were separated into five different controlled classes based on their potential for harm or abuse. Some prescription medications are considered controlled substances and fall into the schedules II – V based on that potential. Not all drugs that require a prescription are considered controlled drugs though. Typically these would be medications used to treat common acute or chronic conditions with very little if any potential for harm or abuse.

Note that not all products available without a prescription are FDA approved. Many vitamins and some dietary supplements and herbal treatments are able to be marketed due to an "all natural" status of their ingredients.

Sometimes an Rx only labeling will appear on the packaging instead of the caution labeling.

Hard copies, meaning the actual paper prescription) should remain on file in the pharmacy. The number of required years, usually 5, is based on the regulations determined by the State Boards of Pharmacy

Prescription Requirements

A prescription order should contain certain pieces of information to be valid or complete. The following information should be present on the script:

* **Name and address of the prescriber**- The written signature will be illegible much of the time. If no printed information is available, feel free to contact the prescriber in order to verify.

* **Name and address of the patient**- The patient's **street address** is required to be on all prescriptions for controlled substances.

* **Patient's date of birth** - Some people have the same name and birthdays can be helpful in determining who's medication you are filling. Also the age of a patient plays a determining factor in correct dosing, especially among children.

* **Date**- Non-controlled prescriptions are only valid one year from date of issue. Controlled substance prescriptions are only valid six months from the written date.

* **Name, strength and dosage form** prescribed.

* **Quantity, volume or weight** prescribed.

* **The directions for use** or "Sig code". The term sig is a Latin abbreviation meaning "take thou"

* **Refill instructions**- if no instructions are given, zero refills are allowed. Note that prescriptions for controlled drugs (III-V) are limited to 5 refills within 6 months but under no circumstances are prescriptions for scheduled II controlled drugs allowed to be refilled.

* **Prescriber's signature** either on dispense as written (DAW) line or generic substitution permitted line. If signed on the DAW line only whatever is written may be dispensed (i.e. brand name) If no difference is notated on call in orders, generic substitution is allowed and the pharmacists notation of the verbal order is sufficient without prescriber signature.

* **DEA number**- this is issued to the prescriber by the Federal Drug Enforcement Administration and is required for all prescriptions of controlled substances.

Prescription Processing

A technician receiving the prescription can begin to screen the **script** for completeness. If a patient's name, address, date of birth (DOB) or prescriber's printed name isn't recorded the technician may begin filling in the blanks by questioning the patient or patient's representative. If other information is missing, it must obtained from the prescriber or prescriber's representative before dispensing. The patient or patient's representative should be questioned each and EVERY time they appear at the window to turn in a new prescription regarding their allergies. Since allergic reactions can happen at any time, with most any medication, this needs to be kept up to date so new prescription medications ordered can be screened against possible allergies the patient may have acquired.

Another area that should be addressed on the receiving end should be **method of payment**; such as insurance, cash or charge. If **third party insurance coverage** (which will be discussed later) is involved, that information must be entered into the system prior to dispensing. Technicians should be familiar with all third party plans that the pharmacy participates in and the co-pays and/or cost that will be due from the patient. Though no technician would ever be expected to have complete knowledge of EVERY insurance plan and its copays, a technician working within a retail pharmacy system should be familiar with the type of prescription drug coverage insurance cards that are accepted there.

Patient medication profiles are maintained for each patient in the computer system's database. Information contained in these profiles would include specific patient information like **name, DOB, address, gender, phone number, insurance information, allergies** and other comments as necessary. This information is stored and updated as changes come about.

The patient profile also contains medications previously dispensed to the patient and these will remain on file for an unlimited amount of time, in most cases. Printed reports can be generated from the patient's profile for a list of medications dispensed during a specific time period (for example, the past year, fiscal year, quarter or month). These types of reports should be distributed to the patient only UNLESS a signed release/consent form has been signed by the patient and that form is on file in the pharmacy. There are various reasons one might be in need of a printed report of this nature.

> Patient profiles within the pharmacy's database of information would include such things as:
>
> * Full name
> * Gender
> * Date of birth
> * Address/Phone
> * Insurance info
> * Allergies

These are some common examples:

* Income Tax purposes as medications may be tax deductible
* Insurance purposes to file a paper claim or proof of payment
* Proof of expense for low income housing or other benefits
* Legal proof that a patient has/has not taken a medication

As new prescriptions are entered into the system, the computer database automatically scans for allergies and drug interactions.

Dispensing Label Requirements

Technicians are often responsible for the data entry of prescription information in order to produce a label for dispensing. There are certain pieces of information that are required to be present on the label. They are as follows:

* Caution: Federal law prohibits transfer of this drug to anyone other than for whom it was prescribed.
* Pharmacy name, address and phone number
* Prescription number
* Prescriber's name
* Quantity or volume dispensed
* Medication name and strength
* Directions for use
* Dispensing Pharmacist's initials (typist's initials sometimes included)
* Refill status
* Date of dispensing

Information that is printed on the label must all be precise but the directions for use must especially be accurate and easily understood by the patient. Abbreviations should be avoided, due to confusion. In the table below see some examples of wording choices. ALWAYS make the route of administration (such as by mouth, rectally, in the ear) very clear to the patient.

Type of medication	Word Choice	Examples
Oral	Adult- take Child-give	Take one tablet Give 1 teaspoonful
External	Apply	Apply to lesions
Suppositories	Unwrap and insert	Unwrap and insert rectally
Ophthalmic/Otic drops	Place, instill or put	Place 2 drops in each eye Instill 3 drops into left ear

Sample Prescription Label

Getwell Pharmacy

555 Hospital Street, Mytown, MS 44499 601-555-1234

Rx 1234567   05-03-2012

Ima Lil Sickly   Dr. Uhl Feelbetter

Many patients have prescription benefit coverage through private or government insurances. When an employee is injured on the job, workman's compensation covers the costs. These payers are referred to as **third party payers** because they are a "third party" involved in the financial transaction between the patient and the pharmacist. Most third party payers have on-line authorization also called **POS** or **point-of-sale**. You can know right then as you fill a prescription if it will be covered by the insurance or rejected for some reason. You can also know right away what the co-payment will be. This is known as **online adjudication**.

The **co-payment** (often called **co-pay** for short) is the portion of the medication cost that is to be assumed by the patient. Sometimes this amount will be set, for example: five dollars for generic prescriptions and twenty dollars for brand-name prescriptions. Other times it will vary based on the cost of the medication. The patient might be expected to pay a certain percentage of the total cost.

Oftentimes, the technician will be the mediator between the patient and the insurance company. If a claim is **rejected**, the technician may call the customer service department of the insurance to assist with the problem. Sometimes, the rejection will be a result of a pharmacy error in data entry. Many times, the patient is no longer eligible on the insurance plan or the prescription may have been recently filled at another pharmacy, among other reasons for rejections.

Perhaps the claim can be repaired and rebilled with a **payable** outcome. If so, the dispensing process can be carried on to the next step. If a payable claim cannot be reached, the script can be kept on hold or sometimes this may be referred to "trouble" on the pharmacy's computer. This is generally where it will stay until either the problem is resolved by working with the insurance company further, by having the patient work with his/her benefits manager to solve the problem or until the patient decides to pay full price for the medication. Computer software varies from pharmacy to pharmacy and one cannot really learn more than the basics of process in training such as this.

After a prescription is deemed fillable, then the next step in the dispensing process can get underway. Preparing the medication for dispensing is one of the jobs most often assumed by the pharmacy technician. Technicians are regularly involved in counting and pouring medications.

The tech is allowed to pull needed **stock** from the shelf. The correct quantity is then poured or counted and placed into a container suitable for dispensing to the patient. The container size selected should be as close to the volume of medication as possible. If it is too large, the patient may think that they are getting shorted. On the other hand, if the container is too small tablets or capsules may be crushed when placing the lid on the container. Also, if the container is too full, it may be easily spilled when opened by the patient.

Auxiliary labels are those small brightly colored labels that are placed on the dispensing container to help patients know more about correctly taking their medication.

A **childproof cap** must be used on the dispensing container according to the **Poison Prevention Act of 1970**. In cases of a patient's desire for **easy-open (non safety caps)**, it must be notated on the back of the script or some other patient information sheet, and should be signed by the patient and kept on file.

After the medication is placed into the dispensing container, the **primary** and **auxiliary** labels can be affixed. These labels need to be situated so that no information is covered. After the prescription is prepared, normally the prescription, the finished product and the stock bottle are assembled together awaiting the pharmacist's verification. Though technicians are generally qualified and able to follow through the filling process (including counting/pouring and labeling) it is the pharmacist who must verify the final product for dispensing.

Most computer systems have NDC identification numbers specific to a particular drug product dispensed, which appear on the label for verifying against the stock bottle. After the pharmacist's verification the stock bottle should be promptly returned to the shelf. Doing so will help to reduce clutter on the pharmacy counter and all the while help reduce the possibility of errors from occurring. Bar-coding technology is being incorporated into the pharmacy workflow more and more these days. This electronic matching process also helps to reduce errors in the dispensing process.

In fact, now many outpatient pharmacies have some type of robotics or automation used in dispensing. Another advancement in technology offers an electronic view of the prescription and also a comparative between what the NDC of the drug used in the data entry for that prescription and the actual physical photo of what the pill/medication should look like.

The finished product is now ready for delivery to the patient. Quite often the dispensing label alone cannot provide all of the needed information for patients. **Auxiliary labels** can usually help fill in the blanks but sometimes even that is not enough. Some computer systems have ability to print out medication information sheets. This will also help the patient know how to use the medication properly. Even still, many patients will need **counseling** by the pharmacist. The **Omnibus Budget Reconciliation Act of 1990** mandated counseling for all new prescriptions for Medicaid patients.

Technicians are prohibited from counseling patients, though they play a key role in identifying patients in need of counseling. Though counseling, due to the demand for pharmacy services is scarce in some locations, has been difficult for pharmacists to provide in the past, many are now seeing some form of relief in that certain services with patients on certain insurance coverages can now be billed through **MTM**'s (**Medication Therapy Management** programs). Medicare Part D has promoted this service with most of their carriers.

Prescription **refills** are handled in a similar manner. The patient may phone in ahead of time for refills without having to wait there in the

Patients are often discouraged from bringing their old bottles back to the pharmacy. HIPAA regulations are strict concerning disposal of anything that has legible patient specific information.

pharmacy. Many pharmacies, especially corporate chains, have an automated voice answering service through which a patient or their representative can enter their prescription number(s) for refills over the phone without ever having to speak directly to a pharmacy staff member. Using this system is a win-win for all involved.

Though they are discouraged in doing so, some patients still bring all of their old bottles into the pharmacy for refilling. Before these bottles can be discarded, the labels must be defaced where personal health information cannot be read or either thrown in with other garbage that is marked for destruction (what sometimes is referred to as the "HIPAA" garbage).

The computer will generate a label for dispensing the refills and automatically subtract a refill from the remaining refills available on the prescription. If a partial fill is done for any reason, the computer will calculate the remaining quantity or volume of medication available.

The transfer of remaining refills on a prescription from one pharmacy to another is allowed in most cases. The receiving pharmacist usually telephones the originating pharmacists for a **verbal copy**. A technician is not allowed to give a "copy" to another pharmacy. This is the responsibility of the pharmacist. In addition, most states prohibit the transfer of prescriptions for controlled substances, even between pharmacies that share the same owner.

Patient contact is the heart of what ambulatory care pharmacy is all about. Technicians are in constant one-on-one contact with their patients. They are the ones who are usually answering the phones, running the cash register, and handling patients' problems such as insurance rejections and charge account situations. Though every day at the pharmacy will certainly not be a glorious day at the park, a technician's good customer service skills can definitely bring repeat business to a pharmacy. However, on the contrary, bad customer service skills can possibly drive a patient into seeking an alternative location for their pharmacy needs.

Oftentimes, a patient will either give their prescription to a technician at the window or speak to a technician on the phone regarding a refill only to return later and pick up their medications and have a technician ring them up at the cash register. All of this the patient may do and never directly encounter a pharmacist in the process. Ambulatory care pharmacy practice can be a stressful, yet rewarding experience for any technician.

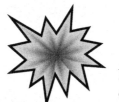

Math Blaster

Pharmaceutical calculations are used to determine the correct dosage amount or the correct amount of a particular ingredient in a compounded medication. There are many different types of calculations needed to correctly prepare and dispense medications. As a result of this fact, we will learn with each practice setting, those calculations that are most commonly dealt with on a routine basis. Please realize that the calculations are universal and all settings will perform most all of the calculations at one time or another.

Ratio and Proportion

Ratio and proportion is a basis for many pharmaceutical calculations. It can be used in several different ways, but particularly in dosing. This setup will become so familiar to you in performing pharmacy calculations because it is perhaps one of the most common foundations of pharmacy math. Ratio and proportion is done using equivalent fractions style configuration. The thing to remember is to keep units in the same place within the two fractions. For instance, in figuring mg/mL, make sure that in both of the fractions, mg are on top as the numerator and mg are on bottom as the denominator.

Hint to remember:

The ratio and proportion technique can be used to calculate many things. Just always remember "what's on top stays on top and what's on bottom stays on bottom. This means if you have mg's on top, mg's go on top on both sides of the equation and so on.

Here is an example:

The pharmacy has in stock albuterol syrup 2mg/5mL. The physician has ordered a dose of 15mL for a patient. What is the strength in mg of the ordered dose? Note that because the given concentration is in mg/mL that the unknown dose is calculated by setting up in the same mg/mL format of
X mg/15 mL.

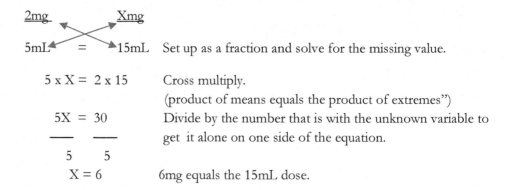

$$\frac{2mg}{5mL} = \frac{Xmg}{15mL}$$ Set up as a fraction and solve for the missing value.

5 x X = 2 x 15   Cross multiply.
(product of means equals the product of extremes")

$$\frac{5X}{5} = \frac{30}{5}$$ Divide by the number that is with the unknown variable to get it alone on one side of the equation.

X = 6   6mg equals the 15mL dose.

The following dosage can be calculated in the same manner as before though this time, the unknown is the volume of the dose and not the strength. Note that because the given concentration is in mg/mL that the unknown dose is calculated by setting up in the same mg/mL format of 375mg/X mL.

The pharmacy has a stock suspension of amoxicillin 250mg/5mL. The dose to be given three times daily is 375mg. Determine the volume of each dose.

$$\frac{250mg}{5mL} = \frac{375mg}{X\ mL}$$

$$5 \times 375 = 250 \times X$$

$$\frac{1875}{250} = \frac{250X}{250}$$

$$7.5 = x \qquad \text{7.5mL equals the 375mg dose}$$

As long as the general rule of "what's on top stays on top" is followed, this type of setup can help determine all manner of comparisons. It is by far, the easiest setup to work out conversions from one unit of measure to another. From time to time, you may be referred back to this area for review if needed.

Total Quantity

Many times it is necessary to perform this calculation type to determine the correct quantity or volume of medication to be dispensed. Very often a prescriber will give a dosing regimen to be followed for a specific period of time and fail to include a quantity or volume of medication to be dispensed. As long as the frequency (i.e. 4 times daily or every 6 hours etc) is given, the dispensed amount can be determined. Simply multiply the doses in each day (determined by frequency) by the number of days and find the amount that is needed to complete the dosing regimen. Take note that "pills" can be counted as 1 each but liquid doses such as teaspoons should be calculated in milliliters since that is how the quantity should be entered into the database.

See the examples below.

Amoxicillin 500mg   i cap tid x 14 days
$$1 \times 3 \times 14 = 42$$

42 capsules will be needed for this regimen.

Cephalexin oral susp 250mg/5mL   250mg qid x 7 days
$$\textbf{5mL} \times 4 \times 7 = 140mL$$
140mL is the total needed.

Prednisone liquid   Take 1 tsp tid x3 days; then

$$\textbf{5mL} \times 3 \times 3 \qquad\qquad = 45mL$$

1 tsp bid x3 days; then

$$\textbf{5mL} \times 2 \times 3 \qquad\qquad = 30mL$$

1 tsp qd x3 days then stop.

$$\textbf{5mL} \times 1 \times 3 \qquad\qquad = 15mL$$
$$+ \rule{3cm}{0.4pt}$$

The sum of all three quantities is: 90mL

as will be the correct dispensing volume.

Days Supply

> When calculating a days supply for a prescription, always figure the maximum amount for each dose and multiply by the most frequent dose allowed by the physician.

Days supply is frequently calculated by technicians, because in most computer systems a days supply must be entered when preparing a label for dispensing.   For refill and insurance purposes, it is required. Here, the calculation involves dividing the total dispensed amount by the number (or volume) of doses per day. When there is a variance in frequency or dosing, always calculate days supply using the largest dose and the shortest frequency.   For instance if 1 or 2 tablets can be taken, it can be assumed that the patient will take 2 tablets. If the dose can be given every 6 to 8 hours, it can be assumed that the patient will take the dose every 6 hours.

Furthermore, any amount of time that does not constitute an entire day is usually dropped rather than rounded off to the nearest whole day. If the calculation ends up that a medication will last 11.7 days, the partial day can be dropped and the actual accepted days supply would be 11 days. See the example below.

Hydrocodone/Acetaminophen   i or ii tablets q46h prn for pain   #32

What is the days supply?   2   x   6   (for a max of 12/day)

$$32 \div 12 = 2.66 \text{ days worth}$$

This would be keyed as a 2 day supply because any remainder would not complete the possible regimen for an entire third day. Any remainder should be dropped.

Insulin Calculations

At times, technicians will have the need to calculate the days supply for insulin. This is slightly different than other days supply calculations because there is a set amount of insulin in each vial and it is measured in units versus the traditional mL or pills in the bottle. When dealing with tablets and capsules, you could simply add or take away tablets to reach the desired days supply of medication. With insulin, it does not work that way. Let's try one and see:

The patient brings you a prescription for insulin. The sig is written for 40 units q am and 20 units q pm. How many days will a 10mL vial last? If we needed to dispense a month's supply (30 days), how many vials must we dispense to the patient?

All insulins are measured in units per ml. The vials are standard size and contain the standard units per vial.

40 + 20 = 60 units per day.   First calculate the total units/day by adding both am and pm doses.

*Each ml contains 100 units of insulin

1000 units ÷ 60 units/day = 16.7 days.   Since there are 1000 units of insulin in each vial, divide for the total days supply.

*Each 10ml vial contains 1000 units of insulin.

1 vial will last this patient 16.7 days   This is counted as 16 days supply. As mentioned before, any portion of an additional day should be dropped.

If we are to dispense a month's supply (30 days) we must give 2 vials for the patient to have enough.

DEA Number Validation

One final calculation coincides with training for the ambulatory care setting. As mentioned earlier, the prescriber's DEA number must be present on all prescriptions for controlled substances. There is a formula that can be used to validate a DEA number. The mantra to keep in mind, especially if something seems fishy on a prescription for a controlled drug... "When in doubt, check it out!"

A DEA number consists of 2 letters and 7 numbers. The first letter is usually A,B or F and the second letter will be the first letter of the prescriber's last name. Some math magic can be performed on the seven numbers to see if the number is valid. Follow the formula given next to learn this technique.

You wish to validate the following DEA number for Dr. Robinson.

AR1634802	First consider the letters. Does the second letter match the first letter in the prescriber's last name? In this case, yes it does. If it does not, you can stop here knowing that the DEA number is invalid.

Although most database systems have built in functions to test the validity of the DEA number, for testing purposes and general knowledge, the tech should be able to perform the validity testing.

$1 + 3 + 8 = 12$	Take the 1st, 3rd & 5th digits and add them together.
$6 + 4 + 0 = 10$	Take the 2nd, 4th & 6th digits and add them together.
$10 \times 2 = 20$	Multiply the sum of the second group by two.
$20 + 12 = 32$	Take this total and add to total of the first group.
	The last digit of the total you arrive at should match the 7th digit of the DEA number.
$32 = 2$	In this case, the DEA number is valid.

Had the last digit been anything other than a 2, it would not have been valid.

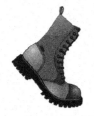

Drill Practice

Complete the following calculations then check yourself in the rear of the textbook. Sometimes a problem may require several steps to solve.

1. The amoxicillin suspension in stock is 250mg/5mL. How much would be given to a patient taking a 100mg dose?

2. A patient is given 22.5 mL per dose of potassium elixir that has a concentration of 10mEq/15mL. What is the strength in mEq of the ordered dose?

3. Cefdinir oral suspension 125mg/5mL is used to fill a prescription with the following directions. 200mg daily for 5 days. What amount in milliliters should be given for each dose?

4. How many tablets will a patient need if he is supposed to take 1 tablet po qid for 30 days?

5. A prescription is dropped off at the pharmacy window. It reads: Lactulose syrup 2 Tbsp tid for 7 days. What amount of lactulose syrup should be dispensed?

6. A prescription for pain patches was ordered. The script directions read: Apply one patch every 72 hours for 15 days. How many patches should be dispensed to the patient?

7. If a patient gets the following prescription from a doctor, how much medication should be dispensed?

    Prelone syrup 5mg/5mL

    Give ii tsp po qid x 3 days, then ii tsp tid x 3 days, then

    ii tsp bid x 3 days, then ii tsp qd x 3 days, then

    i tsp qd x 3 days then stop.

8. A patient presents a script for Prednisone 5mg tablets with the following directions. ii po tid x3 days, then i po tid x3 days, then i po bid x3 days, i po qd x3 days then stop. Calculate the number of tablets needed to fill the order.

9. The physician has written a script for a patient. It reads: Hydrocodone/Acetaminophen 5mg/500mg, i-ii tabs q6h prn #60. What is the days supply calculated for this script?

10. A patient gives the pharmacy a prescription for cephalexin 250mg , ii po tid. If 42 capsules will be dispensed, what will be the days supply for this prescription?

11. How many days will a 8oz bottle of cough syrup last that is dispensed with the following directions? Take 1 or 2 teaspoonsful by mouth every 4 to 6 hours.

12. How many vials of insulin will a patient taking 45 units sq q am and 12 units q pm need for at least 30 days supply? How many days will each vial last?

13. A patient's insulin regimen consists of 70 units each morning and 45 units each evening. How many vials does the patient need each month? How many days will each vial last the patient?

14. Circle the only possible valid DEA# for Dr. Reyes from the choices below.
   a. AD6358217   b. AR6532817   c. BR6358217   d. BD6252716

15. Which of the following is not a valid DEA number for Dr. Franklin Smith?
   a. BS2942729   b. FS7632171   c. AS3724537   d. BS1684681

16. A patients brings the following script to your pharmacy: amoxicillin 400mg po tid for 10 days. You have in stock amoxicillin 250mg/5mL. What is the exact volume of medication you will need for filling this script?

17. The pharmacist takes a call in script from the local clinic. As you are keying the data in for preparing the dispensing label, you must calculate the amount to dispense. The script reads: Cefprozil 200mg po bid for 7 days. The pharmacy only stocks the 125mg/5mL. How much will be needed?

18. You have cephalexin oral suspension 250mg/5mL. The doctor has written for a dose of 150mg. How much will the patient need to take with each dose? How much will the patient need to continue this regimen @ bid for 7 days?

19. How many 20mEq doses can a patient take from a pint bottle of potassium elixir containing 10mEq/15mL?

20. How many 60mg doses are in a 100mL bottle of clindamycin 75mg/5mL?

Drug Training Mission Three

Brand Name	Generic Name	Drug Classification	Primary Indication	Side effects, Warnings, Other
Diflucan	Fluconazole	triazole antifungal agent	treatment or prevention of candidiasis	headache, nausea, abdominal pain, diarrhea, dyspepsia, dizziness
Depakote ER	Divalproex	AntiConvulsant	Epilepsy, Mania associated with Bipolar Disorder and Migraine prevention	May increase risk of hepatotoxicity, teratogenicity and pancreatitis; may also cause somnolence, GI upset and other effects
Viagra	Sildenafil	ED Agent	Erectile Dysfunction	Headache, Flushing
NuvaRing	Etonogestrel/ ethinyl estradiol Vaginal Ring	Contraceptive	Prevention of pregnancy	Vaginitis, headache, upper respiratory tract infection, vaginal secretion, sinusitis, weight gain, and nausea.
Ultram	Tramadol	Centrally acting analgesic	Moderate to Moderately Severe Pain	Dizziness, Nausea & Vomiting, Constipation, Headache, Malaise
Boniva	Ibandronate	Bisphosphonate	Osteoporosis treatment and prevention	Patients should take 1 hour before first food or drink of the day and should not lie down for at least an hour. May cause pain in back or extremities, URI, headache, myalgia, GI upset
Pepcid	Famotidine	Histamine Receptor H_2 Antagonist	Gastric ulcer, esophagitis, Gastroesophageal Reflux Disease (GERD)	Headache, constipation or diarrhea, dry mouth, asthenia, fatigue,
Tenormin	Atenolol	Beta- Blocker	Hypertension	Hypotension, bradycardia, dizziness, nausea
Zantac	Ranitidine	Histamine Receptor H_2 Antagonist	Hypertension, Edema, Hyperaldosteronism	Headache (sometimes severe) constipation or diarrhea, malaise, fatigue

Brand Name	Generic Name	Drug Classification	Primary Indication	Side effects, Warnings, Other
Lidoderm	Lidocaine Patch	Local anesthetic	relief of pain associated with post-herpetic neuralgia	the site of application may develop blisters, bruising, burning sensation, depigmentation, dermatitis, discoloration, edema, erythema, exfoliation, irritation, papules, petechia, pruritus
Tamiflu	Oseltamivir	Anti-viral Agent	Influenza treatment and prevention in patients at least 1 year of age	Nausea and vomiting are common
Avelox	Moxifloxacin	Synthetic Broad Spectrum Anti-Bacterial Agent	Various susceptible infections in adults greater than 18 years of age	May increase risk of tendinitis and tendon rupture in all ages; should not be used in ages less than 18; may also cause nausea, diarrhea, dizziness and other

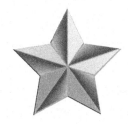

Mission 3 Debriefing

Answer the following questions in assessment of the lessons learned in Mission 3. For best results, repeat the exercise until no questions are missed then move on to the next mission.

1. Having the date on the prescription is not so important because prescriptions do not get too old to be filled?
   a) True
   b) False

2. Which of the following medications carries an indication of pain relief?
   a) Divalproex
   b) Ibandronate
   c) Tramadol
   d) Atenolol

3. The amoxicillin suspension in stock is 125mg/5mL. How much would be given to a patient taking a 75mg dose?
   a) 1.2mL
   b) 0.3mL
   c) 3mL
   d) 8mL

4. Prescription medications are referred to as legend drugs because the Federal law that requires the pharmacy to dispense with a childproof cap.
   a) True
   b) False

5. A patient is given 1 mL per dose of ferrous sulfate elixir that has a concentration of 75mg/0.6mL. What is the strength in mg of the ordered dose?
   a) 125mg
   b) 8mg
   c) 45mg
   d) 100mg

6. A patient using the prescription medication NuvaRing is seeking _____.
   a) Pain relief
   b) A contraceptive
   c) A Blood pressure medication
   d) An infection medication

7. All prescriptions can be transferred by giving/receiving a verbal copy of the prescription via telephone.
   a) True
   b) False

8. Which of the following is not an ambulatory care pharmacy?
    a) Mail order pharmacy
    b) Grocery store pharmacy
    c) Nursing home pharmacy
    d) Internet pharmacy

9. Cefdinir oral suspension 250mg/5mL is used to fill a prescription with the following directions. 300mg daily for 5 days. What amount in milliliters should be given for each dose?
    a) 16mL
    b) 6mL
    c) 7.5mL
    d) 4.2mL

10. Viagra is likely to cause a side effect of flushing.
    a) True
    b) False

11. How many tablets will a patient need if he is supposed to take 1 tablet po qid for 30 days?
    a) 30
    b) 60
    c) 90
    d) None of these

12. Ibandronate should be taken 1 hour before the first food or drink of the day and the patients should not lie down for at least 1 hour after taking the medication.
    a) True
    b) False

13. The _____ is the portion of the prescription costs that is to be assumed by the patient.
    a) Annual deductible
    b) Copayment
    c) Average wholesale price
    d) None of these

14. A prescription is dropped off at the pharmacy window. It reads: Lactulose syrup 2 Tbsp tid for 30 days. What amount of lactulose syrup should be dispensed for the month's supply?
    a) 900mL
    b) 90mL
    c) 2700mL
    d) 600mL

15. A patient gives the pharmacy a prescription for cephalexin 250mg , i po qid. If 56 capsules will be dispensed, what will be the days supply for this prescription?
    a) 14
    b) 56
    c) 7
    d) 28

16. When filling prescriptions, after pharmacists' verification the stock bottle should be promptly returned to the shelf...........Why?
    a) Reduces clutter
    b) Helps to prevent errors
    c) Both A and B
    d) Neither A nor B

17. A prescription for hormone patches was ordered. The script directions read: Apply one patch twice weekly. How many patches should be dispensed to the patient assuming that the pharmacy uses a "4 week" month as a guide?
    a) 4
    b) 8
    c) 56
    d) 16

18. Information that is printed on the dispensing label can be abbreviated to fit because most people understand common pharmacy abbreviations anyway.
    a) True
    b) False

19. If a patient gets following prescription from a doctor, how much medication should be dispensed?   prednisolone syrup 5mg/5mL: Give ii tsp po tid x 3 days, then i tsp tid x 3 days, then i tsp bid x 3 days, then i tsp qd x 3 days, then stop.
    a) 300mL
    b) 36mL
    c) 270mL
    d) 180mL

20. Which of these pairs of medications are H_2 Antagonists?
    a) Depakote ER and Ultram
    b) Lidoderm and Tenormin
    c) Oseltamivir and Moxifloxacin
    d) Ranitidine and Famotidine

21. The financial transaction between the patient and pharmacist often includes benefits paid through another source, such as insurance or workman's compensation. These sources are referred to as third party payers.
    a) True
    b) False

22. The physician has written a script for a patient. It reads: Oxycodone/Acetaminophen capsules 5mg/500mg, i-ii capsules q6h prn #42. What is the days supply calculated for this script?
    a) 5
    b) 3
    c) 10
    d) 7

23. A patient presents a prescription for Tenormin. The patient's provider has written him/her a prescription for a(n) _____.
    a) Anticonvulsant
    b) Betablocker
    c) Analgesic
    d) Antiviral agent

24. A technician is not permitted to complete the labeling for a prescription which involves typing the label, adding the label to the dispensing container and also adding any necessary auxiliary labels to the dispensing container.
    a) True
    b) False

25. A patient presents a script for prednisone 10mg tablets with the following directions. i po qid x 2 days, then i po tid x 2 days, then i po bid x 2 days, i po qd x 2 days then stop. Calculate the number of tablets needed to fill the order.
    a) 40
    b) 100
    c) 20
    d) 200

26. Which of the following drug selections could be written with refills?
    a) C II
    b) C III – V
    c) Non-controlled medications
    d) Only B and C
    e) All of these
    f) None of these

27. Prescriptions for controlled substances are limited to...
    a) 6 refills within 6 months
    b) 11 refills within 12 months
    c) 5 refills within 6 months
    d) 5 refills within 12 months

28. How many vials of insulin will a patient taking 58 units sq q am and 26 units q pm need for at least 30 days supply? How many days will each vial last?
    a) 3 vials needed, each vial lasts 11 days
    b) 2 vials needed, each vial lasts 16 days
    c) 3 vials needed, each vial lasts 12 days
    d) 2 vials needed, each vial lasts 25 days

29. Purchases of behind the counter medications such as cough syrups, syringes and pseudoephedrine products generally requires a specific age for purchasing, a government issued picture ID and sometimes even a signature.
    a) True
    b) False

30. A patient has been diagnosed with an infection. Which of the following medications are they most likely to be prescribed as a result of the findings?
    a) Tenormin
    b) Boniva
    c) Lidoderm
    d) Avelox

31. Taking divalproex may increase the risk of _____.
    a) Hepatotoxicity
    b) Suicidal thoughts
    c) Tendinitis
    d) Blistering skin

32. According to the Poison Prevention Act of 1970, childproof caps must be used on all dispensing containers regardless of patient preference.
    a) True
    b) False

33. Choose the only possible valid DEA # for Dr. Beech.
    a) AB2792485
    b) AD2792845
    c) BB2792845
    d) BB2798959

34. Oseltamivir is indicated for treatment of a variety of bacterial infections.
    a) True
    b) False

35. Moxifloxacin should not be given to which of the following patient age groups?
    a) Less than 1 year of age
    b) Less than 2 years of age
    c) Less than 18 years of age
    d) Over 60 years of age

36. Why is it so important to keep allergy information updated in the computer system?
    a) Allergy information can change at any time.
    b) The system can only screen new prescriptions for allergies if they are entered.
    c) Neither A nor B
    d) Both A and B

37. A technician can counsel a patient regarding their medications if there are questions or concerns?
   a) True
   b) False

38. Generally a hard copy of a prescription is required to be kept on file for at least _____ though this practice is governed by each individual state board of pharmacy.
   a) One year
   b) Two years
   c) Five years
   d) Seven years

39. Customer service skills can help to determine patient satisfaction as well as repeat business.
   a) True
   b) False

40. A patient has been diagnosed with Osteoporosis. Which of the following medications is likely to be prescribed?
   a) Sildenafil
   b) Ibandronate
   c) Divalproex
   d) Oseltamivir

41. All medications requiring a prescription are considered controlled substances.
   a) True
   b) False

42. A patient's profile in the computer system's database contains a list of previously filled medications and insurance information as well as demographics such as address, phone numbers and DOB.
   a) True
   b) False

43. Which of the following is not a valid DEA number for Dr. Vincy Shlameel?
   a) BS1942728
   b) FS7632174
   c) AS3724538
   d) BS2684682

44. A technician can give a verbal copy to transfer a prescription to another pharmacy.
   a) True
   b) False

45. A patient's insulin regimen consists of 50 units each morning and 20 units each evening. How many vials does the patient need each month? How many days will each vial last the patient?
   a) 2 vials needed, each vial lasts 14 days
   b) 3 vials needed, each vial lasts 15 days
   c) 2 vials needed, each vial lasts 15 days
   d) 3 vials needed, each vial lasts 14 days

46. What is the most probably reason for the side effects of blistering, dermatitis, depigmentation or discoloration of the skin when using Lidoderm?
   a) Because it is a drug used to treat neuralgia or nerve pain.
   b) Because of its anesthetic properties.
   c) Because it is in a patch dosage form and applied topically.
   d) Because it is used to treat infection.

47. Which of the following are specifically required and should be present on all prescriptions for controlled substances in addition to any other requirements?
    a) Prescriber's DEA number
    b) Patient's street address
    c) Both A and B
    d) Neither A nor B

48. You have penicillin oral suspension 250mg/5mL. The doctor has written the following script: 100mg qid for 1 week. The patient needs 56mL to complete this regimen.
    a) True
    b) False

49. Processing a prescription through electronic billing and determining if a claim will be paid or rejected is known as online _____.
    a) Adjudication
    b) Orientation
    c) Junction
    d) Distribution

50. The biggest disadvantage of patients using a mail order/internet pharmacy to fill prescriptions is:
    a) Not being able to communicate directly with pharmacy staff
    b) The time involved in receiving the prescriptions
    c) The cost of copayments for using this type of service
    d) None of these

51. Legend drugs require a prescription to acquire.
    a) True
    b) False

52. How many 20mEq doses can a patient take from a 12 oz bottle of potassium elixir containing 10mEq/15mL?
    a) 12 doses
    b) 5 doses
    c) 24 doses
    d) 23 doses

53. Choose the statement below that is true concerning OTC medications.
    a) They can be bought without a prescription "over–the–counter".
    b) They are FDA approved for consumer self-diagnosis and treatment.
    c) They have been tested and are labeled for consumer use.
    d) All of these

54. How many 60mg doses are in a 30mL bottle of diflucan oral suspension 40mg/mL?
    a) 7 doses
    b) 3 doses
    c) 12 doses
    d) 20 doses

55. When a prescriber signs on the DAW or Dispense as Written area, only whatever he/she has written can be dispensed without consultation of the prescriber.
    a) True
    b) False

56. How can missing information on a prescription be determined?
    a) By asking the patient or patient's representative for information such as DOB, address.
    b) By contacting the prescriber for certain information such as DEA number, quantity.
    c) By discussing with the pharmacist for information concerning dosage forms and such.
    d) All of these can be done

57. Auxiliary labels offer additional information to help patients correctly and safely take their medications.
   a) True
   b) False

58. Reports on patient history of prescription drugs in the pharmacy can be used for_____ but should not be release without prior signed patient consent is on file.
   a) Income tax purposes
   b) Insurance purposes
   c) Legal purposes
   d) All of these

59. A patient brings the following script to your pharmacy: clarithromycin 175mg po bid for 7 days. You have in stock clarithromycin 125mg/5mL. What is the exact volume of medication you will need for filling this script?
   a) 7mL
   b) 98mL
   c) 70mL
   d) 140mL

60. A prescription for a controlled substance should have the patient's street address.
   a) True
   b) False

61. A patient's DOB on the prescription can help determine several things including age eligibility for a medication as well as dosage form for the medication.
   a) True
   b) False

62. The pharmacist takes a call in script from the local clinic. As you are keying the data in for preparing the dispensing label, you must calculate the amount to dispense. The script reads: Carbamazepine suspension 200mg po tid for 30 days. The drug is only available in suspension form as 100mg/5mL. How much will be needed?
   a) 900mL
   b) 600mL
   c) 225mL
   d) 450mL

63. What law mandated counseling for all new Medicaid prescriptions?
   a) Controlled Substance Act of 1970
   b) Durham-Humphrey Amendment of 1951
   c) Health Insurance Portability and Accountability Act
   d) None of these laws.

64. How many days will a 6oz bottle of cough syrup last that is dispensed with the following directions? Take 2 teaspoonsful by mouth every 8 hours.
   a) 12
   b) 20
   c) 6
   d) 4

On the following listed items:
Enter a 1 if the information could ONLY be found on a PRESCRIPTION
Enter a 2 if the information could ONLY be found on a DISPENSING LABEL
Enter a 3 if the information could/should be found on BOTH OF THE ABOVE

65. _____ DEA Number
66. _____ Prescriber's Name
67. _____Medication Name and Strength
68. _____ Dispensing Pharmacist's Initials
69. _____ Refill status
70. _____ Federal caution regarding transfer of the prescription medication to other patients
71. _____ Directions for use
72. _____ Prescriber's signature
73. _____ Pharmacy name address and phone number
74. _____ Quantity, weight or volume
75. _____ Prescription number
76. _____ Date

Match the following drugs to their generic names.

77. Tylox   ____ a) ibandronate

78. Viagra   ____ b) famotidine

79. Ultram   ____ c) tramadol

80. Pepcid   ____ d) atenolol

81. Zantac   ____ e) etonogestrel/ethinyl estradiol

82. Lidoderm   ____ f) ranitidine

83. Avelox   ____ g) sildenafil

84. Depakote ER   ____h) oxycodone/acetaminophen

85. NuvaRing   ____ i) divalproex

86. Boniva   ____ j) oseltamivir

87. Tenormin   ____k) lidocaine

88. Tamiflu   ____ l) moxifloxacin

Match the following drugs to their classifications.

89. Oxycodone/Acetaminophen   _____ a) anti-bacterial agent

90. Moxifloxacin   _____ b) anti-viral agent

91. Divalproex   _____ c) local anesthetic

92. Oseltamivir   _____ d) H_2 Antagonist

93. Sildenafil   _____ e) bisphosphonate

94. Lidocaine patch   _____ f) centrally acting analgesic

95. Etonogestrel/ethinyl estradiol   _____ g) H_2 Antagonist

96. Ranitidine   _____ h) contraceptive

97. Tramadol   _____ i) erectile dysfunction agent

98. Atenolol   _____ j) beta blocker

99. Ibandronate   _____ k) opioid analgesic

100. Famotidine   _____ l) anti-convulsant

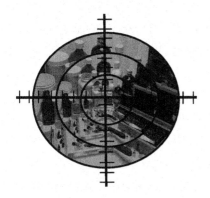

Mission 4:
Institutional
Pharmacy Operations

Mission Objectives

*To recognize the different types of institutional pharmacies.

*To become familiar with aspects of the medication order filling and distribution
   process.

*To understand the various requirements medication orders.

*To become familiar with the equipment used in institutional practice.

*To learn the concept and advantages of unit dosed medications.

*To understand the use and purpose of the Medication Administration Record.

*To become knowledgeable of the major automated dispensing systems.

*To gain baseline knowledge of twelve of the most popular drugs on the market.

*To understand the principles of pharmaceutical calculations used in the
   institutional pharmacy setting including injectable dosage calculations and dosing
   by weight.

Institutional pharmacies serve patients confined to an inpatient setting, meaning that the
patient and pharmacy are generally housed in the same facility. Exceptions to this would be that in
some long-term care facilities, a contracted service is provided and the medications are delivered to
the facility periodically. Various examples of institutional pharmacies are hospitals, mental
institutions, prison infirmaries and long term care (LTC) facilities such as nursing homes, assisted
living or extended care facilities.

Medication Orders

In this practice setting, medications are still distributed on a prescription only basis. The
script just comes in a different form called a **medication order** or **doctor's order**. It must still
include the prescriber's signature or documentation by another member of staff, usually a nurse or
pharmacist, where the prescriber gave a verbal order. An order is not valid unless it contains this
signature or documentation.

Though a prescriber can authorize medications to be ordered by verbal means, he/she
would still be required to review the documented orders and give a signature approval. How often
this is required would be determined by the facility policies. Most hospital institutions require

chartreviews by the prescribers every 24 hours. However, depending upon the type of institution and how often the prescriber makes appearances at that location, the reviews may be extended to one month or longer. The latter would likely be more common in long term care facilities where prescribers may visit monthly or quarterly rather than have the patients come in to their clinics on a regular basis.

A **medication order** is very similar to a written prescription. It is kept in the patient's medical chart which may be a "hard" chart (meaning standard paper forms and documents) or an "electronic" chart (meaning that the facility has/is moving toward an **electronic health record EHR** keeping system). No matter what version of charting a facility has, a copy of medication orders gets sent to the pharmacy for dispensing.

In the institutional setting, one of the greatest differences in receiving medication orders is fact that a phone call or a "call in" prescription is generally NOT accepted. Instead, the pharmacy must receive a direct copy. See examples from the list below of what consists of a **direct copy**.

> *A carbon copy or non-carbon record of the original in the chart
> *A photocopy as from a copying machine
> *A faxed copy
> *An electronic copy via the computer system.

Another big difference to that of the retail or outpatient pharmacy market are **protocols** or **standing orders**. These are routine orders for certain procedures or situations that patients present with that are preapproved by medical staff and/or the **Pharmacy and Therapeutics Committee.** These groups have the authority to make a unanimous decision as to certain labs, medications and other options that can be done or given in a particular circumstance.

Not everything is different between the institutional pharmacy and the ambulatory care setting. Another similarity to outpatient pharmacy would be that the patient's information is kept in a profile in the computer system's database. It is maintained during the length of stay, but because records are kept in the patient's permanent medical chart it isn't necessary to remain on file in the pharmacy for 2 to 5 years. Generally once all information has gone through data processing for billing; it can/will be purged from the active system into a storage system of sorts. Some information contained in the profile is listed at left. Notice the similarities and differences between institutional patient profiles and those of ambulatory care settings.

Unit Dosed Medications

Medications dispensed in the hospital setting are not sent to patient areas in prescription vials or pill bottles as they would be in an outpatient type setting. Instead, they are sent in unit dosed forms. This means that each "dose" that is to be given is packaged in its own bubble or blister pak, sealed dosing cup, oral syringe, vial or injectable syringe or other single dose form.

A medication order should include:

* Patient's name
* Date of birth
* Room number
* Medication name and strength
* Directions for use
* Date and time of order.
* Prescriber's signature or documentation

Profiled information would include:
* Patient's name
* Date of Birth
* Gender
* Weight
* Patient id number
* Date of admission
* Diagnosis
* Allergies
* Medications dispensed

Most often, the medications can be ordered in this individual dose form. However, in the cases where the drug is only available in bulk packaging, there must be some repackaging done on the pharmacy level in order meet the unit dose goal. A closer look at this area of pharmacy practice will be reviewed in Mission 7. Some things are not feasibly packaged in unit dosed forms such as eye drops, ear drops, inhalers and some topical preparations. In these cases, the pharmacy may be able to acquire a small institutional size of the medications.

Most all institutions are now using some sort of **unit dose system.** This has many advantages. It helps reduce **medication errors** because the medication is identified right up to the time it is administered to the patient. Some facilities with the most up to date technologies available have a rolling **computer on wheels (COW)**. It can be pushed right up to the patient's bedside and a nurse is able to bring up the patient's medication profile with all approved medications listed. With a click, a bar-code on the back of the unit dose packaging can be scanned and verified against the active medications that the patient has access to by scanning a barcode on the patient's ID bracelet. This in and of itself is a major technology breakthrough in medication errors at the bedside.

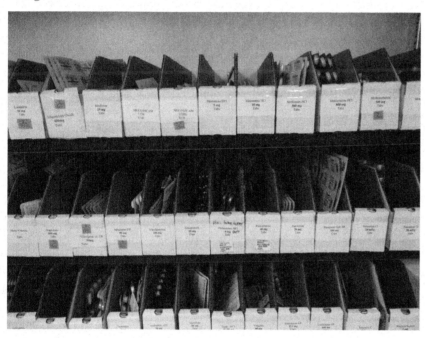

A unit dose system reduces waste and provides a mechanism for more accurate billing, since the patient will only be charged for what he/she receives. Charting is more accurate and convenient because it is done as medications are administered. It is a great mechanism of accountability because the nursing staff must first log in with user name and password and in some cases, a fingerprint, before accessing any patient information.

The **Medication Administration Record (MAR)** serves as the ongoing chart document and is kept with the medication cart. As medication doses are given by nursing staff, they are documented on the MAR. If this is done manually, the nurse will make note of pertinent information such as time and dose and by initialing or signing will confirm that medication has been given. If the healthcare setting has electronic MARs then the notation would be done via a computer system such as the COW. At the patient's time of discharge, the paper MARs or electronically saved information will become part of the patient's permanent record. This takes away the need for additional charting of medication doses during the patient's hospital stay.

Centralized versus Decentralized

There are several types of inpatient pharmacy systems. A **centralized system** is one in that everything is centrally kept in one place. A centralized system is in the pharmacy's main area of the hospital. Here the orders are received, interpreted, filled and distributed back to the nursing unit for administration to the patient. With centralization, only enough doses to provide medications for a set period of time such as 24 hours or 72 hours are sent to and stored on the nursing unit. These medications would be stored in a medication cart with drawers labeled with patient names and their room numbers. A cart exchange would take place at preplanned times in order to bring newly stocked med drawers in exchange for the would be empty ones.

In a **decentralized system** setting, there are several **satellite pharmacies** throughout the entire institution where the actual dispensing process takes place. This type is seen more in larger hospitals where operating the entire pharmacy system from one location would not be convenient. These satellite pharmacies are typically a smaller version of the central pharmacy and their stock usually comes from there. In the satellite pharmacies, an automated dispensing machine stores medications that have been checked and verified by a pharmacist against a "pick list:". Once verified as correct, a technician would then bring the "picked" medications to the nursing unit and place them into the stock of the automated dispensing system.

Due to the nature of specifically needed medications in certain areas, stocking will vary from satellite to satellite. For instance, on the pediatric ward, there will likely be more medications in liquid dosage forms and on the oncology ward where the cancer patients would be housed, there would probably be all manner of pain medications and such as would also be kept in the surgery nursing area.

A combination of both types is becoming more the norm in today's institutional practice settings. This would include areas throughout the hospital where orders are received and interpreted on the nursing ward. In many cases, the orders would be entered in by a technician and verified by a pharmacist before being sent to the larger main pharmacy area where the dispensing function takes place. Perhaps in these cases, medications would be more quickly accessible to nursing staff because numerous items would be loaded already to automated dispensing systems located on the ward.

Instutional Pharmacy Workflow

Technicians are a key player on the institutional pharmacy team. They are usually responsible for making routinely scheduled pick-ups from and deliveries to each nursing unit for new orders and requisitions. As new orders are entered into the system the initial fill of medication is pulled from stock and labeled for delivery. After verification, the delivery to the nursing ward can be made with the next round of deliveries. For routine orders, this happens on a regular repetitive basis throughout the entire shift. However, on occasion there will be STAT orders submitted and these would need to be expedited and filled in front of general orders.

A STAT order would indicate that the medication was emergent and that an immediate response is necessary. Each day a list of all meds needed for each nursing unit is generated. This list is generally referred to as a **pick list**. A technician can use this list to "pick"

meds for each unit and this process is typically called the daily "**cart fill**". The correct number of doses for a 24-hour or other pre-determined period is pulled from stock for medications that are not stored in the automated dispensing systems. These meds along with the meds picked to stock each unit's ADS are verified by the checking pharmacist against the pick list. Once

verified they are ready for delivery to the respective nursing area. Those meds not stocked in the ADS would be placed in the "**cart**" drawers that are labeled for each respective patient. Those meds that are **floor stocked** would be loaded into their areas as well.

Note that though most hospitals DO have some form of automated dispensing process, there are smaller hospitals that still rely on the much older system of the traditional "cart fill". In these cases, an entire cart worth of medications would be brought to the nursing area once it has been verified by the pharmacist. In some instances, there are two sets of carts…one set would be on the nursing unit while the other would be in the pharmacy area being restocked. The swap would occur at a predetermined time by pharmacy and nursing staff and would be kept on a schedule that does not interfere with usual medication administration times. This swap would be called the "**cart exchange**". When the new cart is put in place, the empty one is brought back to the pharmacy to be refilled. Medications that are not feasibly unit dosed, such as eye and eardrops, creams and others would need to be swapped from the old cart to the new before it is returned to the pharmacy.

When patients are admitted to the hospital environment, they may be placed on medication and/or dosages that are not normally for home use. Sometimes, medications are written with an **automatic stop date.** It is often the technician's responsibility to see that these orders do get stopped and are no longer filled and being sent to the nursing unit. A note will usually appear on the pick list when something has been discontinued or stopped. See below for a list of commonly used medications that may be automatically stopped. If a prescriber wishes for a patient to continue on a medication or dosage form that is one with automatic stop date, then the prescriber must reorder or reauthorize it to be filled.

> Chronic medication such as blood pressure meds and others used to treat specific disease states are not generally written with an automatic stop date.

* Strong pain medications, especially CIIs or injectables
* Intravenous fluids and other injectable medications
* Anticoagulant medications
* Special treatment medications such as chemotherapy

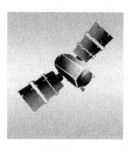

Recon Mission 4:

There are several automated dispensing systems on the market today. Some of the more commonly known ones are Pyxis, Omnicell and Acu-dose. To gather information, do a web search for these products and see what types of systems are on the market. In fact, search not only for printed information such as brochures and product information, but also search for video clips. There are many available for you to view. This will enlighten you on the process and bring a little 3-D to the study of automated dispensing systems.

Technicians are widely used in institutional pharmacy settings. The majority of tasks including data entry and billing, cart filling, drug prepackaging, floor stock, inventory control and department inspections can all be handled by well trained and qualified technicians. Another area that technicians are vital in institutional pharmacy is in the preparation of intravenous admixtures using aseptic technique. We will look at aseptic technique more closely in Mission 5 and the management of inventory and inspections in Mission 7.

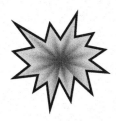

Math Blaster

Here in this mission, a study of dosing calculations for injectables is performed using the previously learned ratio and proportion application. In addition, calculating doses based on a patient's weight is also covered. These processes continue the building blocks of basic pharmacy calculations.

Calculating Injectable Doses

Simple ratio and proportion technique can be used to calculate the amount or strength to administer for injectable doses. As mentioned in the previous mission, this principle is a basis for many pharmaceutical calculations. It can be used in several different ways, but particularly in dosing. Even though previously liquid oral dosages were being calculated, now we will continue to use the equivalent fractions style configuration to figure injectable doses. As a reminder, always remember to keep units in the same place within the two fractions. For instance, in figuring mg/mL, make sure that in both of the fractions, mg are on top as the numerator and mL are on bottom as the denominator.

Here are some examples:

The pharmacy has in stock haloperidol injection 5mg/mL. The physician has ordered a dose of 0.6mL for a patient. What is the mg strength of the ordered dose? First, take a look at the concentration of 5mg/mL. This means that each mL or 1 mL contains 5mg thus it is written 5mg/mL. Note also that because the given concentration is in mg/mL that the unknown dose is calculated by setting up in the same mg/mL format of X mg/0.6 mL.

> Hint to remember:
>
> The ratio and proportion technique can be used to calculate many things. Just always remember **"what's on top stays on top and what's on bottom stays on bottom"** This means if you have mg's on top, mg's go on top on both sides of the equation.

$$\frac{5mg}{(1) mL} = \frac{Xmg}{0.6mL}$$ Set up as a fraction and solve for the missing value.

Cross multiply (top on one side times bottom other side)

$$5 \times 0.6 = 1 \times X$$

$$3 = X$$ 3mg equals the 0.6mL dose.

A properly mixed vial of ceftriaxone injection delivers 100mg/mL. The proper dose per age and weight of the patient is 625mg to be given IM daily for three days. Determine the volume of each dose to administer.

$$\frac{100\text{mg}}{(1)\text{mL}} = \frac{625\text{mg}}{X\text{ mL}}$$ Set up as a fraction and solve for the missing value.

$100 \times X = 625 \times 1$ Cross multiply like before.

$$\frac{100X}{100} = \frac{625}{100}$$ Divide by the number that is with the unknown variable to get it alone on one side of the equation.

$X = 0.625\text{mL}$ 0.625 mL equals the 625mg dose

Dosing by Weight

Another calculation known to institutional pharmacy practice is dosing by weight. Most often dosing by weight calculations are based on a mg/kg/day principle. We can use the mantra of "divide multiply divide" to remember the steps.

There are 2.2 lbs in every kg of body weight.

1kg = 2.2lbs

The first step "divide" is used when converting the patient's weight in pounds to kilograms. So that you understand this process, we can use ratio and proportion to get a better picture.

Say a patient weighs 68 lbs. If we compare the relationship of pounds to kilograms and use equivalent fractions it would look something like this.

$$\frac{2.2\text{lbs}}{(1)\text{kg}} = \frac{68\text{lbs}}{X\text{ kg}}$$ Set up as a fraction and solve for the missing value.

$2.2 \times X = 68 \times 1$ Cross multiply like before.

$$\frac{2.2X}{2.2} = \frac{68}{2.2}$$ Divide by the number that is with the unknown variable to get it alone on one side of the equation.

$X = 30.9\text{kg}$

The child weighs 30.9kg but note that in the end, all that really had to be done was to divide the 68lbs by 2.2 and thus the weight in kg is figured.

With that being said, back to the mantra, "divide multiply divide"…

For pediatric patients being started on phenytoin, the appropriate dose would be 5mg/kg/day in 3 equally divided doses. If a child weighing 68 pounds was placed on this medication, what would be appropriate per dose amount be for dosing this patient 3 times daily?

First, divide...

lbs   lbs/kg   kg

68 ÷ 2.2 = 30.9   First, convert lbs to kg by dividing weight in lbs by 2.2

Next, multiply...

kg   mg/kg   mg/day

30.9 x 5 = 154.5   Next multiply kg by mg/kg to calculate mg/day.

Now, divide again...

mg/day # doses dose

154.5 ÷ 3 = 51.5   Then divide the total by the number of doses within 24 hours.

51.5mg per dose given 3 times daily would be correct.

Be mindful of how the questions you are asked to calculate read. Sometimes you will be given a dose amount and asked to calculate daily usage. Most often, you are given a weight amount and asked to calculate dosage based on that weight and a suggested dosing concentration from the manufacturer.

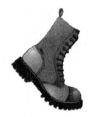

Drill Practice

Complete the following then check yourself in the rear of the textbook.

1. What volume of a 80mg/2 mL tobramycin injection will deliver a dose of 54 mg which needs to be administered?

2. Procainamide injection is ordered at 50mg/kg/day in up 4 divided doses. If a patient taking this medication weighs 154lbs what will the strength of each dose be?

3. Gentamycin is normally given to the average adult at 5mg/kg/day in 3 divided doses. If a patient weighs 132lbs how many milligrams will each dose be?

4. If 640mg dose of medication needs to be given q6h, what volume will need to be drawn from the stock vial if it contains 100mg/mL?

5. A cardiologist has ordered a decrease in dose of a patient's digoxin injection. What volume of a 0.5 mg/2 mL digoxin injection will deliver the newly ordered daily dose of 0.125 mg?

6. A child should receive Tegretol at 20mg/kg/day in 3 equal doses. If the patient weighs 35lbs what will be the strength of each dose?

7. Prochlorperazine is available in a 5mg/mL 10mL Multi-Dose Vial. A physician has ordered 12mg q4h prn nausea post chemotherapy treatments for a patient on the oncology ward. What volume of medication should be administered to achiev e the ordered dose?

8. A 180lb man should receive 10-20mg/kg/day in 2 equally divided doses. What will the range of each dose be? (note: to calculate the range do the problem twice using first the minimum recommended dose and then second using the maximum recommended dose)

9. A 66lb child is to receive 150-200mg/kg/day. What would the range of dosage be per day? (note: this problem is asking for a total daily amount of the medication to be administered so it will be necessary to omit the last "divide" step you learned in the Math Blaster)

10. An elderly patient with advanced infection has been getting vancomycin 1250mg IVPB q6h. If this drug is stocked in 2g/10mL vials, what volume of medication additive should the technician be adding to each piggyback?

11. A 9 year old child is receiving thiamine injection at 25mg IV daily. The pharmacy stocks thiamine in 100mg/mL 30mL Multi-Dose Vials. What amount in milliliters will need to be given for the appropriately ordered dosage?

12. A 58 year old male weighing 165 lbs has been prescribed Amphotericin injection. The recommended dosage is 4mg/kg/day. The once daily approach can be used for the entire amount or the dose can be given in a two equally divided injections. If BID dosing was chosen, what would be the proper amount per recommendations?

13. The physician has recently ordered ampicillin IV for a patient who weighs in at 132lbs. The appropriate dosage is 50mg/kg q6h. How many milligrams would be given each time? (note that the 50mg/kg is the per dose amount)

14. A cancer patient is suffering from nausea after a recent treatment and her physician has approved a one time injection of chlorpromazine. The ordered dose is 40mg IM STAT. If the medication is stocked in a 25mg/mL SDV what volume should be administered to the patient?

15. Trazodone has a recommended dosing of 1.5-2mg/kg/day given in equally divided doses tid. A patient weighing 198lbs has been placed on this medication. What will the range of each dose need to be to remain within recommended manufacturer's guidelines?

16. A drug has been prescribed for a patient at 3g IVPB q6h for infection. It is only available in stock 20g/10mL MDV. What is the appropriate volume amount that should be added to each bag?

17. A onetime dose of pentazocine has been ordered at 20mg IV STAT. Currently the available stock is 30mg/mL 2mL SDV. What volume in milliliters should be withdrawn from the vial to provide the appropriate strength dose?

18. A sedative recommended for children is to be given at 2-6mg/kg/day in 3 or 4 equal doses. Generally recommendations of this nature result in starting with lower doses and titrating up if necessary. The patient has a weight of 88 lbs. What will the range of dosing be if giving TID?

19. A transplant patient has been ordered tacrolimus IV at 0.1mg/kg/day in continuous infusion. If the patient weighs 250 lbs, how many milligrams should be used as an additive?

20. A paramedic on a medical call is needing to give flumazenil injection to a patient in order to reverse benzodiazepine use. The physician orders a maximum dose of 3mg to be given in 0.5mg increments each minute until the patient responds. What is the maximum total volume that can be given if the ambulance stocks the drug in 0.1mg/mL 10mL vials?

Drug Training Chapter Four

Brand Name	Generic Name	Drug Classification	Primary Indication	Side effects, Warnings, Other
Effexor XR	Venlafaxine	Selective serotonin and norepinephrine reuptake inhibitor (SNRI)	Major Depressive Disorder, Generalized Anxiety Disorder, Panic Disorder	May increase risk of suicidal thinking and behavior in children, adolescents, and young adults. headache, asthenia, dizziness, nausea Somnolence, dry Mouth, , decreased sexual function
Nexium	Esomeprazole	Proton-pump Inhibitor	Errosive esophagitis, GERD, gastric ulcer	Nausea, flatulence, abdominal pain, constipation, and dry mouth
Altace	Ramipril	ACE inhibitor	Hypertension	Headache, Dizziness, Asthenia
Zithromax	Azithromycin	macrolide antibiotic	mild to moderate infections	diarrhea/loose stools, nausea, and abdominal pain
Cymbalta	Duloxetine	Selective serotonin and norepinephrine reuptake inhibitor (SNRI)	Depression, Generalized Anxiety Disorder, Diabetic Peripheral Neuropathic Pain, Fibromyalgia	May increase risk of suicidal thinking and behavior in children, adolescents, and young adults. May also cause nausea, dry mouth, constipation, somnolence, hyperhidrosis, headache, insomnia and decreased appetite
Phenergan	Promethazine	Antihistimine, Anti-Emetic	Nausea and vomiting	Drowsiness is the main side effect. This drug should not be given to children under 2.
Namenda	Memantine	NMDA receptor antagonist.	Moderate to severe dementia of the Alzheimer's type	Confusion, constipation, coughing, dizziness, hallucinations, headache, hypertension, pain, insomnia, emesis
Tricor	Fenofibrate	Anti-Cholesterol Agent	Hyper-cholesterolemia; Hyper-triglyceridemia	Abnormal liver function tests, abdominal pain, respiratory disorders

Brand Name	Generic Name	Drug Classification	Primary Indication	Side effects, Warnings, Other
Veetids, PenVK	Penicillin V Potassium	Penicillin Antibacterial	Suceptible strains of infection for various conditions	Patients should be aware of signs/symptoms of reaction to penicillin which could vary. nausea and vomiting, black hairy tongue, abdominal cramping
Prinivil, Zestril	Lisinopril	ACE inhibitor	hypertension	Dizziness, headache, hypotension, pain
Tylenol #3	Acetaminophen w/Codeine	C III Narcotic Combination Analgesic	Mild to Moderately Severe Pain	drowsiness, lightheadedness, dizziness, sedation, shortness of breath, nausea and vomiting
Topamax	Topiramate	Anti-Convulsant	Seizure therapy, migraine headache prevention	depression, insomnia, difficulty with memory or concentration, somnolence, paresthesia, psychomotor slowing, dizziness, and nausea

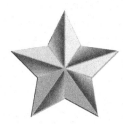

Mission 4 Debriefing

Answer the following questions in assessment of the lessons learned in Mission 4. For best results, repeat the exercise until no questions are missed then move on to the next mission.

1. What must be present on a medication order to validate it?
   a) Prescriber's signature
   b) Verbal order documentation
   c) Either A or B
   d) Neither A nor B

2. A behavioral drug has a recommended dosing of 10-15mg/kg/day given in equally divided doses q8h. A patient weighing 187 lbs has been placed on this medication. What will the range of each dose need to be to remain within recommended manufacturer's guidelines?
   a) 85 – 90mg
   b) 283 – 425mg
   c) 850 – 1275mg
   d) 212 – 318mg

3. The drug promethazine should not be given to which of the following age groups?
   a) Under 2 years of age
   b) Under 6 years of age
   c) Under 18 years of age
   d) Over 60 years of age

4. If a 375mg dose of medication needs to be given q4h, what volume will need to be drawn from the stock 10mL multi-dose vial if it contains 200mg/mL?
   a) 0.9mL
   b) 1.53mL
   c) 1.875mL
   d) 9mL

5. A medication order is very different from a written prescription.
   a) True
   b) False

6. An elderly patient with advanced infection has been getting vancomycin 1750mg IVPB q8h. If this drug is stocked in 2g/10mL vials, what volume of medication additive should the technician be adding to each piggyback?
   a) 0.5mL
   b) 3.75mL
   c) 8.75mL
   d) 9.25mL

7. Typically hospitals require that physicians review charts and sign orders on a daily or 24-hr basis.
   a) True
   b) False

8. Which of the following is likely to be found present in a institutional pharmacy patient's profile?
   a) Admission date
   b) Current and previous medications
   c) Patient weight
   d) Room number and Patient Id number
   e) Patient name and DOB
   f) All of these

9. A drug is available in a 4mg/mL 5mL Multi-Dose Vial. A physician has ordered 7mg q6h prn What volume of medication should be administered to achieve the ordered dose?
   a) 8.75mL
   b) 1.75mL
   c) 1.4mL
   d) 0.57mL

10. Veetids is a macrolide antibiotic.
    a) True
    b) False

11. A pediatric patient weighing 32lbs needs ibuprofen suspension for an increased temperature. The medication can be given at 30mg/kg/day in 4 divided doses. What would be the recommended amount in milligrams per dose?
    a) 435mg
    b) 14.5mg
    c) 108.8mg
    d) 30mg

12. Which of the following pairs of medications are SNRIs?
    a) Nexium and Namenda
    b) Effexor XR and Namenda
    c) Namenda and Cymbalta
    d) Cymbalta and Effexor XR

13. A patient with advanced infection has been getting vancomycin 1700mg IVPB QID. If this drug is stocked in 2g/10mL vials, what volume of medication additive should the technician be adding to each piggyback?
    a) 0.85mL
    b) 1.2mL
    c) 5.7mL
    d) 8.5mL

14. Prescriptions for medications in the institutional setting are required and come in the form of a medication order or a drug order.
    a) True
    b) False

15. Ketorolac therapy is generally started with an injection and then followed by oral dosing. The patient needs a 45mg IM injection and the clinic stocks only 30mg/mL in 2mL SDV. What volume will the correct dose be?
    a) 1.5mL
    b) 3mL
    c) 2mL
    d) 2.5mL

16. A patient's chart may include paper documents in a "hard" chart or it may be kept electronically in an electronic chart system.
    a) True
    b) False

17. A medication order would contain all but which of the following?
    a) Quantity to dispense
    b) Prescriber's signature or documentation of verbal orders received
    c) Medication name and strength
    d) Date and time the order was written or received

18. A 14yr old is receiving thiamine injection at 75mg IV daily. The pharmacy stocks thiamine in 100mg/mL 10mL Multi-Dose Vials. What amount in milliliters will need to be given for the appropriately ordered dosage?
    a) 0.75mL
    b) 0.13mL
    c) 1.3mL
    d) 7.5mL

19. If a patient was diagnosed with Gastroesophageal Reflux Disease (GERD), which of these would likely be prescribed?
    a) Fenofibrate
    b) Esomeprazole
    c) Topiramate
    d) Memantine

20. An institutional pharmacy must keep a patient profile stored in the computer's database for at least two years just as an ambulatory care pharmacy would.
    a) True
    b) False

21. A 0.5mg/kg one time dose of metoclopramide injection is ordered for a small child to assist with small bowel intubation. The child weighs only 22lbs. What is the dose that should be administered?
    a) 5mg
    b) 10mg
    c) 11mg
    d) 50mg

22. Which of the medications below might a patient with high blood pressure be taking?
    a) Altace
    b) Prinivil
    c) Zestril
    d) Any of these

23. A drug has been prescribed for a patient at 3g IVPB q6h for infection. It is only available in stock 10g/10mL MDV. What is the appropriate volume amount that should be added to each bag?
    a) 3mL
    b) 2.5mL
    c) 0.3mL
    d) 0.25mL

24. A prescriber may sign the medication order or give a nurse or pharmacist authorization for a verbal order.
    a) True
    b) False

25. A child is being treated for constipation with lactulose in the recommended 0.125g/kg range with equally divided doses given morning and nightly. The child only weighs 44 lbs so what strength should the appropriate dose be?
    a) 20g
    b) 250g
    c) 2.5g
    d) 12.5g

26. Long term care institutions are likely to have less frequent visits by the prescribing physicians than hospitals do therefore actual signing of orders may extend to once per month or longer.
   a) True   b) False

27. A patient has been ordered an IV medication at 0.1mg/kg/day in continuous infusion. If the patient weighs 126 lbs, how many milligrams should be used as an additive for the once daily medication?
   a) 57.3mg   c) 573mg
   b) 5.73mg   d) 0.6mg

28. When nursing staff has a new order for a patient, they should simply phone the pharmacy to let them know so the medication can be brought to the ward for patient delivery.
   a) True   b) False

29. A patient thiamine injection at 80mg IV daily. The pharmacy stocks thiamine in 100mg/mL 30mL Multi-Dose Vials. What amount in milliliters will need to be given for the appropriately ordered dosage?
   a) 24mL   c) 8mL
   b) 0.8mL   d) 2.4mL

30. A prescription for Tricor has been written for a patient. Most likely the patient is suffering from what condition?
   a) Depression   c) High blood pressure
   b) High cholesterol levels   d) An infection

31. A 146lb 32 year old female needs metronidazole injection IVPB q6h. The manufacturer recommends the drug at 30mg/kg/day in equally divided doses. What mg strength will each dose need to be?
   a) 332mg   c) 66.4mg
   b) 498mg   d) 1992mg

32. Which of the following would be considered advantageous of a unit-dosed system?
   a) Medication errors are reduced   c) Charting by nursing staff is
   b) Billing and accountability are   more efficient
      more accurate   d) All of these are advantanges

33. A pharmacy must receive a direct copy of the order. Which of the following is not considered a direct copy?
   a) non-carbon record   c) fax
   b) phone call   d) photocopy

34. A onetime dose of pentazocine has been ordered at 24mg IV STAT. Currently the available stock is 10mg/mL 5mL SDV. What volume in milliliters should be withdrawn from the vial to provide the appropriate strength dose?
   a) 0.01mL   c) 2.4mL
   b) 0.4mL   d) 12mL

35. Preapproved routine orders for certain procedures or situations that patients present with are called standing orders or protocols.
   a) True
   b) False

36. A pediatric patient weighing 28lbs needs ibuprofen suspension for an increased temperature. The medication can be given at 30mg/kg/day in 4 divided doses. What would be the approximate recommended amount per dose?
   a) 95mg
   b) 13mg
   c) 381mg
   d) 12mg

37. Which of the following is not an institutional pharmacy practice setting?
   a) Hospital inpatient pharmacy
   b) Nursing home pharmacy
   c) Mail order pharmacy
   d) Mental institution pharmacy

38. A script for Tylenol #3 could not be written with refills.
   a) True
   b) False

39. Isoniazide has been ordered for a preventative treatment at 15mg/kg twice weekly. The 101 lb patient should receive what amount in milligrams to achieve the appropriate dose?
   a) 344.25mg
   b) 22.9mg
   c) 688.5mg
   d) 45.9mg

40. Which of the following medications could be used for migraine prevention?
   a) Memantine
   b) Duloxetine
   c) Topiramate
   d) Fenofibrate

41. Satellite pharmacies are present in a _____ setting.
   a) Centralized
   b) Decentralized
   c) Both of these
   d) Neither of these

42. A drug has suggested dosing of 2mg/kg/day with doses split evenly over 6 to 8 hours apart. If a QID approach is used for a patient weighing 286lbs how many milligrams will the patient need for each dose given?
   a) 2.6mg
   b) 260mg
   c) 76.5mg
   d) 65mg

43. Lisinopril and Ramipril are known as _____.
   a) SNRIs
   b) ACE inhibitors
   c) Antibiotics
   d) Narcotics

44. Labetalol IV has been ordered for a 240lb patient and will be given at 0.25mg/kg per manufacturer's recommended guidelines for the loading dose. More can be given every 10 minutes until results are achieved not to exceed 300mg. What should be the correct strength of the initial dose in milligrams?
   a) 109.1mg
   b) 81.9mg
   c) 27.3mg
   d) 42.6mg

96

45. Filling of the automated dispensing systems and/or cart exchanges should take place at times that do not interfere with set administration times that nursing staff uses.
    a) True   b) False

46. A cancer patient is suffering from nausea after a recent treatment and her physician has approved a one time injection of chlorpromazine. The ordered dose is 20mg IM STAT. If the medication is stocked in a 25mg/mL SDV what volume should be administered to the patient?
    a) 2.4mL   c) 1.25mL
    b) 0.8mL   d) 4mL

47. If a medication is ordered STAT, it should considered emergent be filled and delivered as soon as possible.
    a) True   b) False

48. A paramedic on a medical call is needing to give naloxone injection to a patient in order to reverse opiate narcotic use. The physician orders a dose of 0.4mg in repeating increments every 2-3 minutes until the patient responds not to exceed 2mg. What is the maximum total volume that can be given if the ambulance stocks the drug in 0.4mg/mL 5mL SDV vials?
    a) 25mL   c) 1mL
    b) 5mL   d) 0.4mL

49. An alzheimer's patient might be ordered which of the following medications?
    a) Nexium   c) Cymbalta
    b) Namenda   d) Topamax

50. A preventative medication for Tuberculosis exposure has been ordered for a treatment at 15mg/kg twice weekly. The 99 lb patient should receive what amount in milligrams to achieve the appropriate dose?
    a) 675mg   c) 337.5mg
    b) 450mg   d) 45mg

51. A _____ is usually generated around prescheduled times each day or week for use in filling unit dose carts and/or automated dispensing systems.
    a) Med list   c) Automatic stop list
    b) Cart fill   d) Pick list

52. Using the drug Venlafaxine carries a risk of abnormal liver function tests.
    a) True   b) False

53. An injectable medication is ordered at 20mg IV STAT. The drug is available from pharmacy in a 5mg/mL 10mL MDV. What is the correct volume amount to be given?
    a) 40mL   c) 4mL
    b) 20mL   d) 2mL

54. Acetaminophen with codeine is a C IV controlled substance.
    a) True   b) False

55. A drug has been ordered for a 275 lb patient and will be given at 5mg/kg STAT per manufacturer's recommended guidelines. What should be the correct strength of the dose in milligrams?
   a) 2.2mg
   b) 125mg
   c) 312.5mg
   d) 625mg

56. Technicians in the institutional setting may perform all but which of the following tasks?
   a) Replenishing floor stock in automated dispensing systems
   b) Final verification of medication orders
   c) Preparing IV admixtures for admitted patients
   d) Data entry and billing charges

57. If 40mg dose of medication needs to be given q4h, what volume will need to be drawn from the stock 5mL vial if it contains 100mg/mL?
   a) 2mL
   b) 1.25mL
   c) 0.4mL
   d) 4mL

58. For Healthcare systems operating in a decentralized type settings, the exact same medications would be kept in stock no matter of the location in the facility.
   a) True
   b) False

59. An injection is ordered at 30mg/kg/day given in equally divided doses BID. If a patient taking this medication weighs 176lbs what will the strength of each dose be?
   a) 80mg
   b) 2400mg
   c) 240mg
   d) 1200mg

60. Which of the following are often referred to as automated dispensing systems or ADSs?
   a) Pyxis
   b) AccuDose
   c) Omnicell
   d) All of these

61. A sedative recommended for children is to be given at 1-4mg/kg/day in 2 or 3 equal doses. Generally recommendations of this nature result in starting with lower doses and titrating up if necessary. The patient has a weight of 66 lbs. What will the range of dosing be if giving TID?
   a) 10 – 40 mg
   b) 30 – 120 mg
   c) 15 – 60 mg
   d) 20 – 50 mg

62. Medications given to patients in the institutional setting are typically documented on the Medication Administration Record but they must also be documented in the patient's medical chart for long term storage of information.
   a) True
   b) False

63. The COW or computer on wheels serves to reduce medication errors at the bedside.
   a) True
   b) False

64. Which of the following would not likely be issued with an automatic stop date?
    a) Pain meds
    b) IVPB antibiotics
    c) Blood pressure medications
    d) Chemotherapy type medications

65. A 25 year old female weighing 143 lbs has been prescribed an injection. The recommended dosage is 5mg/kg/day. The once daily approach can be used for the entire amount or the dose can be given in a two equally divided injections. If once daily dosing was chosen, what would be the proper amount per recommendations?
    a) 162.5mg
    b) 65mg
    c) 325mg
    d) 143mg

66. What does the acronym MAR represent?
    a) Medical alert research
    b) Medication administration record
    c) Medication administration returns
    d) Medical administration research

67. A child is being treated for bowel disorder with laxative medication in the recommended 0.125mg/kg/day range with equally divided doses given morning and nightly. The child only weighs 33 lbs so what strength should the approximate dose be?
    a) 0.9mg
    b) 1.9mg
    c) 15mg
    d) 1.5mg

68. Who is authorized to accept a verbal order from the prescriber?
    a) Pharmacist
    b) Pharmacy technician
    c) Nurse
    d) Both a and b
    e) Both a and c
    f) A, b and c can all receive them

69. Ketorolac therapy is generally started with an injection and then followed by oral dosing. The patient needs a 50mg IM injection and the clinic stocks only 60mg/mL 2mL vial. What volume will the correct dose be?
    a) 0.8mL
    b) 1.2mL
    c) 1.6mL
    d) 2.1mL

70. The physician has recently ordered an IV medication for a patient who weighs in at 132lbs. The appropriate dosage is 20mg/kg q8h. How many milligrams would be given each time?
    a) 1200mg
    b) 60mg
    c) 380mg
    d) 400mg

71. In healthcare systems using a centralized pharmacy approach, all orders are received, interpreted, filled and delivered from a central location with minimum doses being distributed to nursing units for dispensing.
    a) True
    b) False

72. An anticonvulsant is recommended for children to be given at 3-5mg/kg/day in 3 or 4 equal doses. Generally recommendations of this nature result in starting with lower doses and titrating up if necessary. The patient has a weight of 44 lbs. What will the range of dosing be if giving QID?
   a) 15 – 20mg
   b) 15 – 25mg
   c) 25 – 33mg
   d) 20 – 25mg

73. A pharmacist is generally responsible for making routine pick-ups and deliveries from nursing wards.
   a) True
   b) False

74. A drug has suggested dosing of 0.02mg/kg/day with doses split evenly over 6 to 8 hours apart. If a TID approach is used for a patient weighing 286lbs approximately how many milligrams will the patient need for each dose given?
   a) 1.2mg
   b) 0.8mg
   c) 130mg
   d) 1.3mg

75. An injectable medication is ordered at 20mg IV. The drug is available from pharmacy in a 4mg/mL 10mL MDV. What is the correct volume amount to be given?
   a) 50mL
   b) 0.2mL
   c) 5mL
   d) 0.5mL

76. Allergic reactions to penicillin could include but not be limited to nausea and vomiting, black hairy tongue and severe abdominal cramping.
   a) True
   b) False

Match the following drugs to their generic names.

77. Topamax   _____ a) venlafaxine
78. Effexor XR   _____ b) ramipril
79. Prinivil   _____ c) duloxetine
80. Altace   _____ d) esomeprazole
81. Tricor   _____ e) azithromycin
82. Cymbalta   _____ f) promethazine
83. Phenergan   _____ g) topiramate
84. Namenda   _____ h) penicillin V potassium
85. Zithromax   _____ i) memantine
86. Veetids   _____ j) acetaminophen with codeine
87. Nexium   _____ k) lisinopril
88. Tylenol #3   _____ l) fenofibrate

Match the following drugs to their classifications.

89. Venlafaxine
90. Esomeprazole
91. Ramipril
92. Azithromycin
93. Duloxetine
94. Topiramate
95. Acetaminophen with codeine
96. Lisinopril
97. Penicillin V Potassium
98. Promethazine
99. Fenofibrate
100. Memantine

_____ a) NMDA receptor antagonist
_____ b) SNRI
_____ c) Penicillin antibacterial
_____ d) Anti-Cholesterol agent
_____ e) ACE inhibitor
_____ f) Macrolide antibiotic
_____ g) SNRI
_____ h) Narcotic combination analgesic
_____ i) Anticonvulsant
_____ j) ACE inhibitor
_____ k) Anti-emetic
_____ l) Proton pump inhibitor

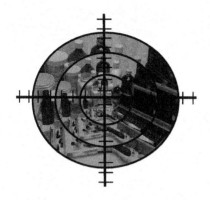

Mission 5: Sterile Product Preparation

Mission Objectives

* To define and understand the principles of using Aseptic technique.
* To gain knowledge of the proper use and function of the Laminar Flow Workbench.
* To become familiar with special procedures used in preparing sterile chemotherapy
    products and other hazardous substances.
* To learn the abbreviations and locations of various routes of administration for parental products.
* To learn correct procedures for using Personal Protective Equipment.
* To gain knowledge of the most commonly used intravenous fluids and their abbreviations.
* To gain baseline knowledge of twelve of the most popular drugs on the market.
* To understand the principles of calculating flow rates for intravenous fluids including drops per minute, milliliters per hour, total volume and total run time.

Parental injections bypass the gastrointestinal tract, since they are injected directly into body tissues and do not have to be absorbed through the normal digestive process. Some parental routes of administration are not injection dependent and those routes do not have to maintain sterility. Some good examples of this type of administration are nasal preparations and oral inhalers. Others are either injectable dependent routes or that which requires sterility (such as ophthalmic preparations) The products that are being administered through injectable dependent routes or that are ophthalmic in nature must be **sterile** and free of **pyrogens** and **particulate matter**.

The injectable **routes of administration** come in handy when the patient is unable to take meds by mouth for whatever reason. It's also used in treatments where rapid absorption is essential, beneficial and possibly even emergent. Medications given by parental injection will normally have a quicker onset of action. This route can be used to correct fluid and electrolyte imbalances and can be used to provide nutrition when food cannot be taken by mouth or feeding tube. The parental route can also be effective for local anesthetic effects in surgery. Those were some advantages of parental medications, but like most everything else, this route also has its disadvantages. It is much more costly and takes more time to administer. Using the parental route also requires the use of trained personnel. It can be painful for the patient and stopping all the effects, if necessary, after administration is extremely difficult. Infection becomes a risk due to the skin puncture; therefore, using aseptic technique is definitely a must.

Routes of Administration

There are several different routes of parental injections. Of these, **subcutaneous (SQ), intramuscular (IM)** and **intravenous (IV)** are the most commonly used. In subcutaneous injections, the solution or suspension is injected underneath the skin. This route usually has a slower onset. The maximum volume that can be injected subcutaneously is 2mL. Patients, especially insulin-dependent diabetics, can easily be taught how to self-administer this type of injection.

Note: Any meds to be given by intrathecal injection must be preservative free.

The intramuscular route is quicker acting than the subcutaneous route. It is injected deep into a large muscle mass, like the buttocks, thighs or upper arms. Up to 2.5mL can be given in this form of injection. The biggest disadvantage to IM injections is the pain that is normally associated with it. The intravenous route is the fastest option where parental administration is concerned because medication is introduced straight into the bloodstream. This is best for medicines that are irritating because they are quickly diluted. The IV route is not as limited to volume as are the other parental routes.

Other routes of administration are intradermal or into the skin and intraarterial or into the artery. We refer to injection into bone marrow space as intraosseous and into the spinal cavity as intrathecal. Intraperitoneal means making injection into the peritoneum or abdominal area.

There are three ways that IV medications can be administered.

* Bolus or initial dose sometimes referred to as a loading dose.

* Continuous infusion

* Piggyback or intermittent infusion

An initial dose, often referred to as a **bolus dose**, can be injected into the vein over a short period of time. This will normally be written **IVP** for **intravenous push**. It is generally used for a small volume. Not all medications can be "pushed". In the package insert for a medication, information regarding this type of use can be found. If, in fact, it can be given in this manner, specific instructions will be included.

Another type of IV injection is called a **continuous infusion**. This involves a larger volume of solution spread over a longer administration time at a constant flow rate. Continuous infusions are primarily for volumes that are 500mL or greater, or for fluid orders that are to run at a specific flow rate for an extended length of time.

There can also be **intermittent infusions** that are delivered through the same administration set to avoid another needle stick. A secondary set will be spiked into a "Y" port on the primary line. These types of infusions are usually smaller volumes of 500mL or less to be given over a shorter time span than the continuous infusion. It's commonly known as a **piggyback** and will usually be written **IVPB**. Antibiotic injections giving using the IV route are commonly piggybacked. Because they are given with additional fluids running at the same time, the IV antibiotics are further diluted and are less irritating to the vein.

Filtration

Filtration is the method of sterilization most commonly used in a pharmacy. There are many pore sizes for filters, but to be a **sterilizing filter**, the pore size mustn't be larger than 0.2 microns. This type of filtration is used whenever a glass bottle or other intravenous fluid container is used. Because this type of container requires a vented administration set, the air passing into the container is filtered in order to remain sterile. Larger pore size filters can be used in solution clarification.

> Oftentimes this will be referred to as 0.22 microns and can be considered the same.

When withdrawing solution from an **ampule,** a 5-micron filter needle is acceptable to prevent tiny glass fragments from entering the final product for injection. Further study will be done regarding ampules and their usage as the mission continues.

There are other sterilization methods like cold and heat sterilization. Cold sterilization uses chemicals like ethylene oxide gas and radiation. Heat sterilization uses pressure and steam, as in an **autoclave**, which is hot enough to sterilize or kill any organisms.

As a note to the limitations of **filterization** and **sterilization**, a 0.2-micron filter will not remove **pyrogens**; furthermore, pyrogens will not be destroyed by autoclaving. Any product that contains pyrogens must be discarded. When commercially prepared sterile products are used and the preparation is done using aseptic technique there is very little concern for the presence of pyrogens on the part of the pharmacy technician.

> A pyrogen is a substance that causes fever.

The concern for pyrogens comes in when a sterile product is being compounded from a non-sterile one and this mainly occurs at the manufacturing level. A great extent of testing is done at this level to ensure that the sterile parental products and the containers that these products are being packaged in are able to remain pyrogen free. Routine inspections and maintenance checks are done to assert that pyrogen free products are being produced.

Aseptic Technique and Laminar Flow

The term "**aseptic technique**" is simply the means of manipulating sterile products without contamination. Bacteria are everywhere and can be very easily transferred to the product from the supplies, environment or the personnel. Maintaining good practices when preparing sterile products will uphold the sterility of the finished product. Sterility, simply put, is the state of being free from all microorganisms.

Compounding sterile products should take place in a **class 100 area** and normally, this area is only found within the **Laminar Flow Workbench (LFW)** often referred to as the "hood". A class 100 area contains no more than 100 particles 0.5 micron or larger for each cubic foot of air. The Laminar flow workbench or "hood" is a confined area that moves filtered air with uniform velocity along parallel lines. The airflow passing through the filter will be moving at least 90 feet/minute and can be horizontal or vertical. The difference will depend on what types of medications are being prepared and this will be expanded on later in this

mission. A **HEPA** filter on the hood removes the particles that are larger than 0.5 micron in size.

The Laminar Flow Workbench (LFW) should be located away from traffic, doors, vents or anything else that is moving faster than 90 feet/minute or the current speed of airflow within the hood that is being used. Any air currents that are greater than the velocity of the airflow from the HEPA filter can introduce microorganisms into the hood. Quick movement in and out of the hood and especially talking, coughing and sneezing while working in the hood are some examples of incidences where there could be a disturbance in airflow.

The **buffer area**, often called the **"clean room"** is the site where the Laminar Flow Workbench (LFW) is located. This area is second in cleanliness only to the area inside the hood. Since overcoming the 90-feet/minute velocity of the airflow underneath the hood is very easily done, this buffer area should be an enclosed area away from the other normal operations in the pharmacy. It should be as isolated as possible away from doors and windows and out of the general pass through flow of traffic.

The biggest source of contamination in a clean room is the personnel. A person that is sitting releases 100,000 particles per minute. That number is increased tremendously when the person moves at a rate of 2mph, which is the average normal walking speed. It jumps to approximately 5 million particles per minute. All personnel should be taught to reduce the introduction of contaminates to the buffer area.

In fact, it is of the utmost importance to deter the addition of particles released into the area. Therefore, no cardboard packaging, paper towels or other high particle count materials are recommended to be in this area. All hand washing, gowning and unpackaging supplies are done in the anteroom area to help reduce the number of particles in the buffer area.

The **anteroom** is an area of higher cleanliness than normal, but not as clean as the buffer area. This area is used for decontaminating supplies, equipment, and personnel. Here in the anteroom, cases of IV fluids, commonly used medication stock may be stored. As these medications and fluids are moved into the clean room area, they are unboxed and carried in to be stored on dust-free shelving. Also in the anteroom, the **Personal Protective Equipment (PPE)** and other back stock of sterile supplies such as needles and syringes may be found. Again, this type of stock is unpackaged and moved into the clean room to be stored in such a manner as to resist the collection of dust particles.

Decontamination of personnel including hand washing and donning of PPE in preparation for working in the buffer area takes place in the anteroom as well.

The first step in doing this is being properly scrubbed and gowned. The technician should remove all jewelry before scrubbing to ensure the hands and wrists are cleaned thoroughly. He/She should also don a knee length gown that ties in the back, head cover, shoe covers and sterile gloves. The gown sleeve cuffs will go inside the gloves. Before entering the hood, the technician should put on a facemask. (This entire garb is the personal protective equipment or PPE) Frequently, the gloves needed to be rinsed with a foam or gel sanitizing agent, such as 70% isopropyl alcohol when entering and re-entering the hood. For this reason, the foam or gel sanitizer would be kept near the hood area.

Once the technician has prepared him/herself the Laminar Flow Workbench (LFW) must also be prepared. The hood should be cleaned at least once per shift even if it is not going to be used during that entire shift. It should also be cleaned before and after use. Depending on the type of hood being cleaned and used, the technique may vary slightly. It is always best to go by the manufacturer's suggested guidelines in order to maintain the cleanest environment possible in which to prepare the sterile products. The statements below are general knowledge and should be considered as such.

The blower should remain on at all times. If it is turned off it must remain on at least 30 minutes prior to use. The LFW must be cleaned with a 70% Isopropyl Alcohol or other sanitizing agent using a non-shedding wipe. Most of the time, a 4 x 4 gauze is used. A new wipe or clean area of the wipe should be used when beginning to clean a new surface area of the hood. There are numerous references to the exact technique used in cleaning a Laminar Flow Workbench. The general knowledge would be to work in a manner that is from the top downward and from the filter area outward so that all possible contaminants are being moved down and out away from the HEPA filter area. Listed below are general knowledge statements that are used in most incidences.

> A good rule of thumb when cleaning the LFW is to work outward and downward away from the HEPA filter. There are many conflicting resources on this subject and the given suggestions are just guidelines. Always use the recommended methods for cleaning that are given by the manufacturer.

* First, the bar should be wiped down thoroughly.
* Second, the top of a horizontal hood or back of a vertical hood should be cleaned using overlapping strokes moving in an "S" motion moving outward or downward away from the HEPA filter.
* The sides of the hood are cleaned beginning at the back of the hood closest to the filter and wipe from top to bottom overlapping strokes working outward as you go along. Some resources suggest cleaning from back to front with overlapping strokes working downward along the side wall. Either method would serve the same purpose.
* The other side should be repeated in the same fashion.
* Last, the hood's work surface is also thoroughly cleaned starting at the back of the hood, closest to the filter using side-to-side continuous motion working to the front outer edge.

As mentioned before, when working in the LFW, aseptic technique is a must. Items placed inside the hood for use (i.e.: vials, bags, amps) should be wiped properly beforehand, unless they are packaged in a protective over wrap. In this case, you should open the over wrapped items at the edge of the hood and place them inside.

When opening syringes and needles, the split ends of the package should be peeled back in a "banana" like fashion with the opening of the package aimed at the

HEPA filter. Oftentimes, a technician could continue to use the same syringe providing that the medication and its concentration remain the same. A needle will become dull after a few punctures through the tough rubber stopper injection ports and may need to be changed. If extra needles are expected to be needed, they should remain with packaging intact until just before use. These extra needles should be placed within the first 6 inches of the hood until needed.

Manipulations inside the hood should be done so that all critical sites remain in constant airflow. A **critical site** is any opening or pathway between the environment and the sterile product. Depending on which type of hood is being used, the manipulations would be done differently in order to avoid blocking this afore mentioned airflow.

Items in a **Horizontal Laminar Flow Workbench (HLFW)** are placed on either side of the critical work area. This critical work area should stay in direct airflow at all times. A technician should avoid a permanent block in airflow between the HEPA filter and any part of the sterile product being compounded. The hands should not become stagnant directly behind any critical site so as to block the flow of air. If airflow is blocked even for a few moments, the particle count in that particular area may be increased and make the product potentially unsafe.

In the Horizontal LFW hood the air intake runs along the lower outer edge of the work surface as well as up the sides of the hood. The air is pulled behind the HEPA filter where it can be cleaned. As air is pulled through the filter, it is sent horizontally across the work surface. Much of it is quickly recirculated and as a result, the longer the motor on the hood is running, the cleaner the air inside the work area gets. The rest of the air is introduced into the room air surrounding the hood.

Even the Vertical LFW hood has the same mechanisms. The difference is the location of the HEPA filter. In the vertical hood, the filter is in the top of the hood instead of the back.

When preparing sterile products containing hazardous materials, you should use the **Vertical Laminar Flow Workbench (VLFW)** or a **Class II Biological Safety Cabinet (C2BSC)** suitable for working with hazardous substances. Since the airflow is not directed toward the preparer, it is much safer when working with hazardous materials. When working with this type of hood, items should be placed so that work may be performed without remaining directly above any critical sites.

The air intake on a Vertical LFW hood is from the top. Air is pulled from the room through intake vents and sent through the HEPA filter. As it enters the work surface area, it continues downward. As it reaches the work surface, it is quickly reabsorbed and sent back through an exhaust HEPA filter before being ventilated to the outside of the building without being recirculated. The ventilation may be hard ducted to the outside or connected with other ventilation systems used within the hospital setting that vent to the outside of the building. Ultimately, there is NO recirculation of any of the contaminated air.

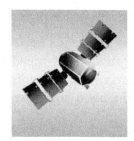

Recon Mission 5:

There are several manufacturers of Laminar Flow Workbenches and Isolator glove boxes on the market today. To gather information, do a web search for these products and see what types of systems are available. It may also be helpful and beneficial to seek out images for sterile product preparation supplies and processes, especially diagrams. In fact, search not only for printed information such as brochures and product information, but also search for video clips. There are many available for you to view. This will enlighten you on the process and bring a little 3-D to the study of sterile product preparation.

Supplies

Some basic items you will be using when working in the LFW are:

* Intravenous solutions
* Needles
* Syringes
* Ampules
* Vials

Intravenous solutions can be supplied in several different types of containers. A **flexible plastic bag** is the most commonly used container. There are two main types of plastic bags used for IV solutions. The most popular one is the **polyvinyl chloride (PVC)** bag. This type of bag is autoclavable and therefore its demand is typically higher. The major alternative to PVC is **Ethylene vinyl acetate or (EVA)** This type of rigid plastic container is much less flexible than the PVC but is better suited for those medications that need to be stored in the freezer or perhaps that would react with the plastics in the PVC.

Regardless of the type of plastics used in the container, a **non-vented set** will be used and it will be known as a closed system because no air enters the container. The bag will simply collapse, as the volume of fluid gets lower. This type of container has two ports. One port is designed to accept the spike of the administration set and the other port is where the medication additives are injected.

Some medications must be delivered in a glass container. When a glass container is used, it is likely because the medication may react with the plastic in the more commonly used types of containers and alter its effectiveness in some way. Because these glass containers require the use of a **vented administration set**, they are referred to as a **semi-closed system**, because the air entering the container is filtered. The air vent contains a 0.2-micron sterilizing filter, which lets air pass through but stops bacteria from getting inside the container. The closure is a solid rubber stopper with a thinner spot in the center for spiking the set and injecting additives. This is the more modern use of the glass container.

Below in the table is a list of regularly used intravenous solutions and their common names to pharmacy and nursing staff.

Medication Name and Percent strength	Commonly Used Names and abbreviations
0. 9% Sodium Chloride	Normal Saline, NS , NaCl
0.45% Sodium Chloride	Half Normal, ½ NS
0.225% Sodium Chloride	Quarter Normal, ¼ NS
5% Dextrose in Water	D5W,D_5W
10% Dextrose in Water	D10W,D_{10}W
5% Dextrose/ 0.9% Sodium Chloride	D5 Normal or D5 NS
5% Dextrose/ 0.45% Sodium Chloride	D5 ½ Normal or D5 ½ NS
5% Dextrose/ 0.225% Sodium Chloride	D5 ¼ Normal or D5 ¼ NS
Lactated Ringers	LR or "Ringers"
5% Dextrose/ Lactated Ringers	D5LR

The larger the gauge number is, the smaller the needle and its bore size will be. Likewise, the smaller the number is, the larger the needle and its bore size will be.

Needles come in many different sizes that are measured by both length and gauge, which measures the thickness in diameter. Lengths can vary from 0.5 inches to 1.5 inches. 28 and 29 gauge needles are the smallest and 13 gauge is the largest. Those needles smaller than 20 gauge are typically used to administer injectable medications. When preparing sterile products, the 18 and 16 gauge needles are most helpful. Their large bore allows for quicker withdrawals and transfers of medications.

Basic parts include the **hub, shaft, bevel, bevel heel** and **tip**. A needle's critical sites are the **hub** and **tip**, but for safety's sake, there really should not be any handling of the needle other than to attach it to the syringe. The needles will be packaged in a sterile paper over wrap or enclosed in a sterile plastic covering. Once opened, there is never any reason to wipe the needle with alcohol as with other supplies. If it is accidentally touched, it should be removed, discarded and replaced with a fresh needle.

The needle's hub, the colored part, is what actually makes contact with the syringe and allows attachment. Though the needle's length and gauge may vary, the hub size is standard and will fit any standard syringe tip. Typically, these are color coded for the various gauges and the colors will likely match with the gauge size regardless of what manufacturer's product is used. See the images below to gain a better idea of the variance in needle gauge size, lengths and hubs.

110

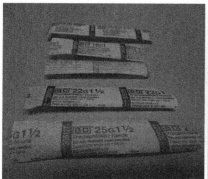
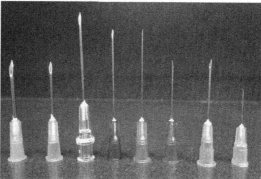

Syringes also come in many sizes ranging from 1mL to 60mL. You need to select the one closest to the volume of fluid you'll be working with. The larger the syringe, the further the **calibration markings** are apart. Therefore it would be more difficult to get an accurate measurement in smaller increments on a larger syringe. Syringes will also come in a sterile outer wrap. This may be paper or hard plastic container. The basic parts of a syringe are the **barrel, plunger, piston,** and the **tip** of the syringe. The top edge of the barrel has a lip on it called the **top collar**. The plunger also has a small lip on it known as the **flange**.

There are two types of syringe tips. One is a **slip tip**, in which the needle fits snuggly on to the syringe. The other type is a **luer-lock** that is threaded to allow the needle to be screwed onto it. The luer-lock syringe type should be used whenever hazardous medications are being prepared. The barrel will be marked according to the calibration of volume it holds. When drawing and measuring fluids in a syringe, the final edge of the piston should be aligned with the calibration mark that corresponds with the volume you desire.

When attaching the needle to the syringe, point the over wrap opening toward the HEPA filter and peel the paper back like a banana. Hold the needle with the thumb and finger of one hand. While holding the syringe in the other hand, twist off the tip of the syringe and push or twist the needle onto it. After the needle is attached you are ready to withdraw your solution. Place the prepared syringe in the Laminar airflow while you prepare your ampule or vial for withdrawal. See the images below to gain a better idea of the variance in syringe size.

A good rule of thumb when choosing syringe sizes is to try and never go more than double the size of volume you need. For instance, if you needed only 10mL of volume, you would not want to use larger than a 20mL syringe.

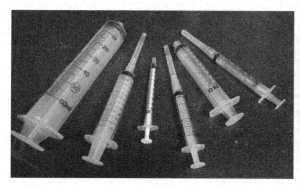
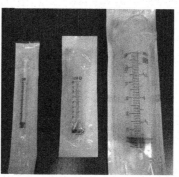

When using an **ampule**, the solution is always ready to use so there will be no need to further dilute before withdrawal. A 5-micron **filter needle** is needed to filter out tiny glass fragments from your final preparation. The filter needle should only be used in a single direction. This means that if the filter needle is used when pulling the solution from the ampule, then it would need to be changed before adding the withdrawn solution into the final product.

It could be also used in the second step where the fluid is withdrawn from the ampule with a regular needle and then a filter needle is put in place to filter the solution as it is pushed into the final product. A good philosophy on this subject is that if glass fragments never get into the syringe, then they cannot possible get into your final product. Therefore, best practices would filter the solution as it is pulled from the amp.

When breaking the ampule, wrap in a sterile 4x4 gauze so that the tiny fragments of glass will have less chance of cutting you.

The amp should have been properly wiped with 70% isopropyl alcohol, as all other items, before being placed in the hood so there is no need to rewipe it down. Hold the amp in an upright position and slightly tap the neck to bring all the solution to the bottom. Pointing the amp away from the HEPA filter (preferably toward the side of the hood) hold it so that both thumbs are directly on either side of the weakened neck and apply pressure as if breaking a pencil in half. The top should snap off with ease because the neck is scored. Be careful not to touch the broken edge with your hands or the tip of the needle. The critical site on an ampule is the **neck**. It should always be in continuous Laminar airflow.

Take the syringe with **filter needle** attached and the amp you have prepared and hold both at an angle with the tip of the needle in the solution at all times. It helps to have the lumen of the needle in the downward position so that the entire contents can be easier withdrawn. Pushing against the flange of the plunger slowly draw the solution from the amp until the desired amount is withdrawn. After this you'll need to pull back slightly on the plunger to allow for pulling all the solution that is left in the needle through the filter. Change from the filter needle before injecting the solution into your final preparation.

Withdrawing solution from a **vial** is slightly different. A vial is a small plastic or glass container, which is closed with a rubber stopper covered with a flip top seal. It must have air injected into it to place **positive pressure** inside the vial before you're able to withdraw the contents because it is a closed system with a vacuum. Before entering the vial, remove the flip top seal by popping it off with your thumb. Wipe the rubber seal with the 70% isopropyl alcohol to clean before entering the vial with the needle.

Pull back on the plunger to the volume of solution you'll be withdrawing to fill the syringe with air. Hold the vial with one hand while using your other hand to maneuver the syringe. At about a 60-degree angle,
place the needle against the rubber stopper with the heel of the bevel and the lumen facing upwards. Apply slight pressure and as you enter the vial, raise the syringe to a vertical position. Invert the vial and slowly inject the air from the syringe. Pull the bevel down close to the rubber stopper and keep the tip in the solution so as to withdraw the solution and not just air.

Adjust the plunger to the appropriate amount you desire and then turn the vial back over. Be careful not to interrupt the airflow to the **rubber stopper** of the vial, as this is its critical site. Slowly remove the syringe from the vial and inject the solution into your final preparation.

Sometimes the contents of the vial are in a dry powder form and must be **reconstituted**. This is done in the same way as above, with the exception of injecting fluid rather than the air. The fluid you inject will give enough positive pressure inside the vial that you'll be able to withdraw what you need after mixing and dissolving.

Hazardous Sterile Products

When working with hazardous substances in Vertical Laminar Flow Workbench or Class 2 Biological Safety Cabinet, there are special precautions that must be taken. The pharmacist in charge should validate that any and all personnel working with hazardous substances are properly trained to do so in order to both protect the pharmacy staff as the medication is being prepared and also the patient who is to receive the medication being prepared.

The pharmacy staff that is expected to handle these hazardous substances should be provided with all safety information as well as to make sure the staff understands their rights as workers under the OSHA "Right to Know" law. The general practice of preparing hazardous sterile products has similarities as other non-hazardous products. Aseptic technique is still a must and additionally, other things must be considered as well.

Here are some additional considerations for handling hazardous substances in the hood.

* Gloves should be disposable, latex and powder free.
* The knee length gown should not be worn outside the designated area.
* A respirator should be worn when not protected by VLFW or BSC.
* Appropriate goggles should be worn for eye protection.
* Work inside the hood should be performed on a plastic backed paper liner which should be changed with each batch of medications and disposed of properly.
* Luer-lock syringes and intravenous sets should be used.
* Syringes should not be filled more than ¾ full.
* Venting devices should be used to avoid aspiration and aerosolization.
* Final products should be dispensed with IV administration sets attached and in a sealed plastic bag labeled as hazardous.
* Any spills require the use of a "spill kit" for cleaning.

Regardless of the type of sterile product being prepared, it must be verified by a pharmacist prior to dispensing or delivery to the patient. The pharmacist will check the preparation for accuracy in calculations, particulate matter, and also that the label is correct.

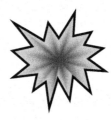

Math Blaster

Because of today's technologies, manual calculation of flow rates is almost a thing of the past. In most cases these days, the administering nurse would simply key the information desired into an automated pump system and the electronic device would calculate and set the correct rate of flow. But for testing purposes and knowledge of this task, we must learn to figure rates of flow the old fashioned way.

Many times you will be asked to figure the milliliters per hour (mL/hr) rate for a particular iv admixture. It may be necessary to determine the total run volume or number of bags to be dispenses. Oftentimes, you will need to figure the rate in drops per minute (gtts/min). In either case the math is easy once you know where to put your numbers.

Milliliters per Hour

To answer the mL/hr part of a question, simply divide the total volume by the number of hours it is to run. Lets try some examples:

A 500mL bag of iv fluids is supposed to run over 6 hours. What is the flow rate in mL/hr?

total   run

volume ÷ time =   mL/hr

500mL ÷ 6 hours = x mL/hr

83.33 = x mL/hr

83 mL/hr would be the correct flow rate because you must round to the nearest drop. (hint: 5 or above rounds up, 4 or less rounds down)

A doctor has ordered 1200mL of 0.9% sodium chloride to run over 8 hours. What is the flow rate in mL/hr?

total   run
volume ÷ time   =   mL/hr

1200mL ÷ 8 hours = x mL/hr
               150 = x mL/hr

150 mL/hr would be the correct flow rate.

Total Run Volume

Sometimes it may be necessary to determine the total volume needed for a specific flow rate and time frame. This would allow the correct number of bags to be sent to the patient location to be administered as ordered. Follow along with the examples below.

If a continuous infusion is to run at 80mL/hr for 12 hours, what is the total volume that will be administered to the patient?

flow   x   run   =   total
rate   time   volume

80mL x 12 hours = 960mL

It may also be necessary to calculate the proper number of fluid bags to dispense for the appropriate volume. Try this one.

How many 500mL bags will need to be dispensed if a patient is receiving a continuous infusion at 100mL/hr for 24 hours?

flow   x   run   =   total
rate   time   volume

100mL x 24 hours = 2400mL

Logically thinking, it will take 5 bags if they are 500mL size to cover the entire volume that has been ordered. If necessary, the total volume could be divided and evaluated that way.

total   ÷ bag   = number of
volume   size   bags dispensed

2400mL ÷ 500mL = 4.8 bags

Since a partial bag cannot be dispensed, the amount will simply need to be upped to the next whole bag. 4.8 bags becomes 5 bags.

Let's try one more of those:

A patient is to receive a continuous infusion at a rate of 80mL/hr for 20 hours. If the nurses are using 500mL stock bags, how many will it take to complete the entire volume that has been ordered for the patient?

flow   x   run   =   total
rate   time   volume

80mL x 20 hours = 1600mL

Logically thinking, it will take 4 bags if they are 500mL size to cover the entire volume that has been ordered. If necessary, the total volume could be divided and evaluated that way.

total   ÷ bag   = number of
volume   size   bags dispensed

1600mL ÷ 500mL = 3.2 bags

Not to be confused with rounding, the amount would simply go up to the next bag number. For instance if 3.2 bags were needed, this number could not simply be "rounded": to the nearest whole number of "3" bags because that would not be enough. Instead, it would need to be upped to the next number of 4 bags. 3.2 bags becomes 4 bags dispensed.

Drops Per Minute

If the calculation is more detailed and you are to figure gtts/minute a total volume of fluid and a run time will be given. Additionally, there will possibly be a specific size administration set used. In this case, you would use the following format to set it up. Remember to use this set up each and every time you calculate gtts/minute. However, if you are not prompted to calculate gtts/minute then this calculation "chart" will be of no benefit to you and should not be used.

total # mL	# gtts	1 hour		gtts
total time in hours	1 mL	60 minutes	=	minute

Notice that mLs and hours will cancel each other out leaving only drops/minute. Multiply across both above and below the line. Then divide the total number of drops on top by the total number of minutes on bottom to get your answer.

> If there is no mention of specific administration set size with calibration of drops per mL given, you will use the standard setting of 60 gtts/mL when calculating flow rates.

D_5W /0.45% NS 1000mL is to be administered over 6 hours using a set that delivers 40gtts/mL. Calculate the flow rate in gtts/min.

$$1000 \times 40 \times 1 = 40,000$$

1000mLs	40 gtts	1 hour		40,000 gtts
6 hours	1mL	60 minutes	=	360 minutes

$$6 \times 1 \times 60 = 360$$

$40,000 \div 360 = 111.11$ gtts/min (don't forget to round)

111 gtts/min would be the correct flow rate for this regimen.

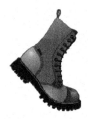

Drill Practice

Complete the following then check yourself in the rear of the textbook.

1. An i.v. infusion order is written for 1000mL of D_5W/0.45%NS to run over 12 hours. The set you have will deliver 15gtts/mL. What should the flow rate be in gtts/min?

2. 1500mL of Lactated Ringers solution is to be given over 16 hours. Determine the number of mL/hr.

3. Determine the flow rate in gtts/min if 50mL of mannitol is to be administered over a 2-hour period.

4. What is the flow rate in mL/hr if 1000mL of NS is to be given over 6 hours and the set delivers 20gtts/mL?

5. What is the total volume that will be needed if D5W is to run at 80mL/hr for 24 hours?

6. How many 1-liter bags (1000mL) will be needed if a patient is getting Normal Saline continuous infusion at a rate of 125mL/hr for 24 hours?

7. An i.v. infusion order is written for 1000mL of Lactated Ringers to run over 14 hours. What should the flow rate be in mL/hr?

8. How many 500mL bags will be needed if a patient receives D5W at 50mL/hr for 16 hours?

9. A patient is to receive 1000mL of D5/0.45 NS with 20 mEq of KCl IV solution over 24 hours. Give the flow rate in gtts/min.

10. An i.v. infusion order is written for 1000mL of D_5W/0.225%NS to run over 12 hours. The set you have will deliver 40gtts/mL. What should the flow rate be in mL/hr?

11. 1000mL of dextrose solution is to be given over 10 hours. Determine the number of gtts/min if the set your using delivers 10gtts/mL.

12. Determine the flow rate in mL/hr if 250mL is to be administered over a 4-hour period.

13. What is the flow rate in gtts/min if 1000mL of D5NS is to be given over 8 hours and the set delivers 40gtts/mL?

14. What is the total volume that will be needed if D5LR is to run at 125mL/hr for 6 hours?

15. How many 1-liter bags (1000mL) will be needed if a patient is getting Half Normal Saline continuous infusion at a rate of 100mL/hr for 16 hours?

16. An i.v. infusion order is written for 1000mL of LR to run over 14 hours. The set you have will deliver 40 gtts/mL. What should the flow rate be in gtts/min?

17. How many 1L bags will be needed if a patient receives NS continuous infusion at 125mL/hr for 10 hours?

18. What is the flow rate in mL/hr if 500mL of D_5W is to be given over 8 hours and the set delivers 20gtts/mL?

19. A patient has been ordered to receive 1000mL of D5NS to run over 8 hours. What should the flow rate be in mL/hr?

20. An i.v. infusion order is written for 1000mL of D_5W/0.45%NS to run over 12 hours. The set you have will deliver 15gtts/mL. What should the flow rate be in gtts/min?

Drug Training Chapter Five

Brand Name	Generic Name	Drug Classification	Primary Indication	Side effects, Warnings, Other
Tessalon Perles	Benzonatate	Non-Narcotic Oral Anti-Tussive Agent	Symptomatic Cough Relief	sedation, headache, dizziness, GI upset
Vitamin D	Ergocalciferol	Calcium Regulator	Hypoparathyroidism, Rickets	Earlier side effects may include weakness, headache, nausea and vomiting, diarrhea, dry mouth, bone pain and metallic taste. Patients should be monitored for long term side effects such as abnormal kidney function.
Flomax	Tamsulosin	Prostate Alpha 1 Agonist	Benign prostatic hyperplasia	Abnormal ejaculation, pain, upper respiratory symptoms, diarrhea, dizziness
Microzide	Hydrochlorothiazide	Diuretic	Hypertension (alone or combined with other agents)	Weakness, hypotension, GI upset, anemia, vertigo, parasthesia, headache, impotence
Risperdal	Risperidone	Anti-Psychotic Agent	Schizophrenia, Bipolar Mania	Elderly patients with dementia-related psychosis treated with antipsychotic drugs are at an increased risk of death
Adipex P	Phentermine	C IV anorectic agent	Weight loss in exogenous obesity	Primary Pulmonary Hypertension, Palpitations, GI issues
Robaxin	Methocarbamol	Skeletal Muscle Relaxant	Acute painful musculoskeletal conditions	Edema, fever, headache, bradycardia, hypotension, dyspepsia, nausea and vomiting, drowsiness
Proscar	Finasteride	Androgen Inhibitor	Symptomatic benign prostatic hyperplasia	Asthenia, hypotension, edema, dizziness, decreased libido, rhinitis, abnormal ejaculation, impotence and abnormal sexual function

Brand Name	Generic Name	Drug Classification	Primary Indication	Side effects, Warnings, Other
Allegra	Fexofenadine	Antihistamine	Seasonal allergic rhinitis	Drowsiness , cough, vomiting and other GI upset
Plavix	Cyclopidogrel	Aggregation Inhibitor (Anti-Platelet)	Treatment of recent Myocardial Infarction or stroke, peripheral arterial disease or acute coronary syndrome	Hemorrhage is the most probable side effect. Caution should be used when combining therapy of this drug and aspirin or other medications with anti-coagulant properties
Pravachol	Pravastatin	Lipid-lowering agent	Hypercholesterolemia	Musculoskelatal pain, GI upset, upper respiratory disturbances
Concerta	Methylphenidate Extended Release	C II CNS Strimulant	Attention Deficit Hyperactivity Disorder (ADHD)	Upper abdominal pain, decreased appetite, headache, dry mouth, nausea, insomnia, anxiety, dizziness, weight decreased, irritability

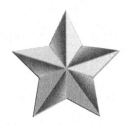

Mission 5 Debriefing

Answer the following questions in assessment of the lessons learned in Mission 5. For best results, repeat the exercise until no questions are missed then move on to the next mission.

1. Which of the following needle sizes makes the largest bore?
    a) 29
    b) 23
    c) 20
    d) 16

2. An i.v. infusion order is written for 1L of Lactated Ringers solution to run over 12 hours. What should the flow rate be in gtts/min?
    a) 72 gtts/min
    b) 83 gtts/min
    c) 102 gtts/min
    d) 8 gtts/min

3. Benzonatate is indicated for weight loss.
    a) True
    b) False

4. Patients, especially insulin-dependent diabetics, can easily be taught how to self-administer this type of injection.
    a) Subcutaneous injections
    b) Intramuscular injections
    c) Intravenous injections
    d) Intraarterial injections

5. 2000mL of ½ NS with 20mEq potassium chloride solution is to be given over 16 hours. Determine the number of mL/hr if the set delivers 40gtts/mL.
    a) 83 mL/hr
    b) 125mL/hr
    c) 68 mL/hr
    d) 42 mL/hr

6. A schizophrenic patient might be taking which of these medications?
    a. Flomax
    b. Robaxin
    c. Plavix
    d. Risperdal

7. Parental injections must _____.
    a) be sterile
    b) be pyrogen free
    c) contain no particulate matter.
    d) all of these

8. Determine the flow rate in gtts/min if a 250mL bag containing 1g vancomycin is to be administered over a 2-hour period with a set delivering 40gtts/mL.
   a) 125 gtts/min
   b) 42 gtts/min
   c) 60 gtts/min
   d) 83 gtts/min

9. Which pairs of medications are indicated for benign prostatic hyperplasia?
   a) Methocarbamol and cyclopidogrel
   b) Tamsulosin and finasteride
   c) Pravastatin and hydrochlorothiazide
   d) Phentermine and tamsulosin

10. Items placed inside the hood for use should be wiped properly beforehand, even if packaged in a protective over wrap.
    a) True
    b) False

11. What is the total volume that will be needed if D5W is to run at 80mL/hr for 8 hours?
    a) 800mL
    b) 640mL
    c) 960mL
    d) 460mL

12. Laminar Flow Workbench (LFW) should be cleaned _____
    a) at least once per shift.
    b) before and after use.
    c) Only when it's used and dirty
    d) All of these
    e) Both a and b
    f) Neither b nor c

13. Which of the following pairs of drugs are controlled substances?
    a) Adipex P and Concerta
    b) Allegra and Robaxin
    c) Plavix and Pravachol
    d) Microzide and Allegra

14. An i.v. infusion order is written for 1500mL of Lactated Ringers to run over 24 hours. What should the flow rate be in gtts/min if the set delivers 60gtts/mL?
    a) 63 gtts/min
    b) 42 gtts/min
    c) 83 gtts/min
    d) 125 gtts/min

15. Hand washing, gowning and unpackaging supplies are done in the buffer area to help reduce the number of particles in the anteroom.
    a) True
    b) False

16. A patient is to receive 2L of D5LR solution over 24 hours. Give the flow rate in mL/hr.
    a) 63 mL/hr
    b) 83 mL/hr
    c) 100mL/hr
    d) 125mL/hr

17. Which of the following is not an advantage of using injectable routes of administration?
    a) Can be used when PO meds cannot be taken,
    b) provides rapid absorption for a quicker onset of action.
    c) can be painful
    d) can provide nutrition if necessary

18. A patient taking Allegra probably is suffering from what condition?
    a) Hypertension
    b) Cough
    c) Seasonal allergies
    d) High cholesterol levels

19. Which subcutaneous injections, the solution or suspension is injected into the skin.
    a) True
    b) False

20. What is the flow rate in gtts/min if 1000mL of NS is to be given over 10 hours and the set delivers 40gtts/mL?
    a) 67 gtts/min
    b) 100 gtts/min
    c) 60 gtts/min
    d) 83 gtts/min

21. How many 1L bags will be needed if a patient is getting Normal Saline continuous infusion at a rate of 100mL/hr for 24 hours?
    a) 1 bag
    b) 2 bags
    c) 3 bags
    d) 4 bags

21. The biggest sources of contamination in a clean room are the supplies.
    a) True
    b) False

22. Which of the following medications could not be phoned in or prescribed with refills?
    a) Adipex P
    b) Proscar
    c) Plavix
    d) Concerta

23. 1000mL of dextrose solution is to be given over 10 hours. Determine the number of gtts/min if the set your using delivers 10gtts/mL.
    a) 17gtts/min
    b) 10gtts/min
    c) 14gtts/min
    d) 15 gtts/min

24. Which of the following statements are true concerning preparation and delivery of hazardous.
    a) Gloves should be disposable, latex and powder free.
    b) Appropriate goggles should be worn for eye protection.
    c) Any spills require the use of a "spill kit" for cleaning.
    d) All of these

25. A patient in need of a "fluid pill" may be prescribed _____.
    a) Tamsulosin
    b) Cyclopidogrel
    c) Hydrochlorothiazide
    d) Finasteride

26. An i.v. infusion order is written for 1000mL of NS to run over 12 hours. The set you have will deliver 40 gtts/mL. What should the flow rate be in mL/hr?
    a) 25mL/hr
    b) 56mL/hr
    c) 63mL/hr
    d) 83mL/hr

27. A class 100 area contains no more than 100 particles _____ or larger for each cubic foot of air.
   a) 0.2 micron
   b) 0.5 micron
   c) 4 micron
   d) 5 micron

28. Which of the following may have been prescribed for a patient who has suffered from a recent stroke?
   a) Plavix
   b) Proscar
   c) Pravachol
   d) Adipex P

29. How many 1L bags will be needed if a patient receives Ringer's solution at 125mL/hr for 10 hours?
   a) 1 bag
   b) 2 bags
   c) 3 bags
   d) 4 bags

30. All but which of the following can introduce microorganisms into the hood.
   a) Quick movements
   b) Cleaning the hood properly
   c) Excessive talking and head movement
   d) coughing and sneezing into the hood

31. A critical site is any opening or pathway between the environment and the sterile product.
   a) True
   b) False

32. If the blower on the hood is turned off it must remain on at least _____ prior to use.
   a) 15 minutes
   b) 30 minutes
   c) 45 minutes
   d) 60 minutes

33. What is the flow rate in mL/hr if 500mL of D_5W is to be given over 8 hours and the set delivers 40gtts/mL?
   a) 63mL/hr
   b) 42mL/hr
   c) 25mL/hr
   d) 22mL/hr

34. Phentermine is classified as a(n)_____.
   a) Antihistamine
   b) Anorectic agent
   c) Aggregation inhibitor
   d) Antitussive

35. Which of the following statements is true concerning pyrogens?
   a) A 0.2-micron filter will not remove pyrogens.
   b) Pyrogens will not be destroyed by autoclaving.
   c) Any product that contains pyrogens must be discarded.
   d) All of these statements are true.

36. How many 500mL bags will be needed if a patient receives D5W at 50mL/hr for 12 hours?
   a) 1 bag
   b) 2 bags
   c) 3 bags
   d) 4 bags

37. The anteroom is the site where the Laminar Flow Workbench (LFW) is located.
    a) True
    b) False

38. The drug Pravachol is indicated for patients who have _____.
    a) BPH
    b) Hypothyroidism
    c) ADHD
    d) Hypercholesterolemia

39. Parental injections do not bypass the gastrointestinal tract and must be absorbed through the normal digestive process.
    a) True
    b) False

40. An i.v. infusion order is written for 1000mL of D_5W ½ NS to run over 12 hours. The set you have will deliver 15gtts/mL. What should the flow rate be in mL/hr?
    a) 21mL/hr
    b) 83mL/hr
    c) 63mL/hr
    d) 56mL/hr

41. When patients are taking ergocalciferol, they should be monitored for long-term side effects such as _____.
    a) Weight loss
    b) Abnormal kidney function
    c) Hemorrhage
    d) Dementia related psychosis

42. Determine the flow rate in gtts/min if 100mL is to be administered over a 2-hour period.
    a) 25 gtts/min
    b) 50 gtt/min
    c) 75 gtts/min
    d) 100 gtts/min

43. The anteroom is used for decontaminating _____.
    a) supplies
    b) equipment
    c) personnel
    d) All of these

44. Which of the following is not a disadvantage of using parentally injected medications.
    a) more costly
    b) take more time to administer
    c) infection becomes a risk
    d) provides anesthesia when needed

45. A patient has been ordered to receive 1000mL of D5NS to run over 8 hours. What should the flow rate be in mL/hr?
    a) 100mL/hr
    b) 56mL/hr
    c) 83mL/hr
    d) 125mL/hr

46. A pyrogen is a substance that causes fever.
    a) True
    b) False

47. A vented administration set filter should be _____ to ensure the sterility of the air entering the glass container.
    a) 0.2 micron
    b) 0.5 micron
    c) 4 micron
    d) 5 micron

48. Which of the following types of syringes should be used whenever hazardous medications are being prepared.
   a. Slip tip
   b. Luer-lock
   c. Either a or b
   d. Neither a nor b

49. Which of the following is classified as a skeletal muscle relaxant?
   a) Fexofenadine
   b) Cyclopidogrel
   c) Methocarbamol
   d) Methylphenidate

50. Which route has the fastest onset?
   a) Subcutaneous injections
   b) Intramuscular injections
   c) Intravenous injections
   d) Intradermal injections

51. What is the flow rate in gtts/min if 500mL of D5NS is to be given over 6 hours and the set delivers 40gtts/mL?
   a) 56 gtts/min
   b) 63 gtts/min
   c) 83 gtts/min
   d) 125 gtts/min

52. With some medications, an initial dose of a small volume can be "pushed" or injected into the vein over a short period of time. This will normally referred to as_____
   a) Continuous infusion
   b) Bolus dose
   c) Piggybacked infusion
   d) None of these

53. When withdrawing solution from an ampule, a _____ filter needle is acceptable to prevent tiny glass fragments from entering the final product for injection.
   a) 0.2 micron
   b) 0.5 micron
   c) 4 micron
   d) 5 micron

54. Compounding sterile products should take place in a _____ area
   a) Class 100
   b) Class 1000
   c) Class 10,000
   d) Class 100,000

55. An i.v. infusion order is written for 1000mL of D5¼NS to run over 8 hours. The set you have will deliver 40gtts/mL. What should the flow rate be in gtts/min?
   a) 100 gtts/min
   b) 42 gtts/min
   c) 83 gtts/min
   d) 63 gtts/min

56. When preparing sterile products containing hazardous materials which of these below should be used?
   a) Vertical Laminar Flow Workbench
   b) Class II Biological Safety Cabinet
   c) Either a or b
   d) Neither a nor b

57. How many 500mL bags will be needed if a patient is getting ½ NS continuous infusion at a rate of 100mL/hr for 16 hours?
   a) 1 bag
   b) 2 bags
   c) 3 bags
   d) 4 bags

58. Which of the following statements are false concerning decontamination and donning of PPE?
    a) The technician should properly scrub and gown him/herself.
    b) The technician should remove all jewelry before scrubbing.
    c) A knee length gown that ties in the back should be worn.
    d) The gloves should go under the gown sleeve cuffs.
    e) Head covers, shoe covers, facemasks and sterile gloves should be worn.
    f) All of these are true.

59. The HEPA filter on a Laminar Flow Workbench removes the particles that are larger than _____ in size.
    a) 0.2 micron   c) 4 micron
    b) 0.5 micron   d) 5 micron

60. What is the total volume that will be needed if D5LR is to run at 125 mL/hr for 6 hours?
    a) 722mL   c) 750mL
    b) 21mL   d) 1750mL

61. A larger volume of solution spread over a longer administration time at a constant flow rate is commonly called _____.
    a) continuous infusion.   c) loading doses
    b) intermittent infusions   d) any of these

62. Whenever a glass bottle of intravenous fluids or medications is dispensed, it requires a _____ administration set.
    a) Non-vented   c) Either a or b
    b) Vented   d) Neither a nor b

Number the statements 63-66 below in the order they should go when cleaning the hood. For instance, the first step should get number 1, the next step, number 2 and so on.

63. _____ The top or back should be cleaned using overlapping   strokes

64. _____ The bar should be wiped down thoroughly.

65. _____ The work surface is cleaned working outward from the filter using side-to-side continuous motion

66. _____ The sides of the hood are cleaned from back to front, top to bottom overlapping strokes working outward from the filter.

Match the intravenous solutions below with their common abbreviations.

67. 0. 9% Sodium Chloride   ____a) D$_5$W
68. 5% Dextrose in Water   ____b) ¼ NS
69. 5% Dextrose/0.9% Sodium Chloride   ____c) D5 ½ NS
70. 0.225% Sodium Chloride   ____d) D5LR
71. 10% Dextrose in Water   ____e) ½ NS
72. Lactated Ringers   ____f) D5 NS
73. 5% Dextrose/0.45% Sodium Chloride ____g) NS
74. 0.45% Sodium Chloride   ____h) D$_{10}$W
75. 5% Dextrose/0.225% Sodium Chloride____i) D5 ¼ NS
76. 5% Dextrose/Lactated Ringers   ____j) LR

Match the following drugs to their generic names.

77. Concerta   _____ a) benzonatate
78. Tessalon Perles   _____ b) tamsulosin
79. Plavix   _____ c) methocarbamol
80. Flomax   _____ d) phentermine
81. Proscar   _____ e) methylphenidate
82. Risperdal   _____ f) pravastatin
83. Adipex-P   _____ g) ergocalciferol
84. Robaxin   _____ h) hydrochlorothiazide
85. Allegra   _____ i) cyclopidogrel
86. Microzide   _____ j) fexofenadine
87. Pravachol   _____ k) risperidone
88. Vitamin D   _____ l) finasteride

Match the following drugs to their classifications.

89. Benzonatate   _____ a) CNS Stimulant
90. Ergocalciferol   _____ b) Lipid lowering agent
91. Tamsulosin   _____ c) Aggregation inhibitor
92. Hydrochlorothiazide   _____ d) Antihistamine
93. Risperidone   _____ e) Androgen inhibitor
94. Phentermine   _____ f) Skeletal muscle relaxant
95. Methylphenidate   _____ g) Anoretic agent
96. Pravastatin   _____ h) Antipsychotic agent
97. Cyclopidogrel   _____ i) Diuretic
98. Fexofenadine   _____ j) Prostate Alpha-1 agonist
99. Finasteride   _____ k) Calcium regulator
100. Methocarbamol   _____ l) Antitussive agent

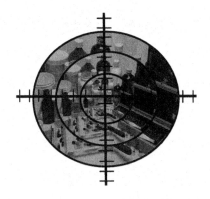

Mission 6:
Basics of Compounding
in the Pharmacy

Mission Objectives

*To understand the reasons for compounding in the pharmacy setting.

*To identify the various dosage forms of medications.

*To become familiar with special equipment used in preparing compounded products.

*To define bulk and extemporaneous compounding.

*To become familiar with preparation of a compounding log.

*To learn and understand the formulas used to perform compounding calculations.

*To perform calculations used in compounding including allegations and concentrations and dilutions

*To gain baseline knowledge of twelve of the most popular drugs on the market.

Prior to 1950 about 80% of medications were compounded on site in the pharmacy setting. A physician would prescribe a medication and the "druggist" would simply mix the desired ingredients accordingly and prepare the ordered medication. However, during this era came the birth of mass manufactured medications as well as the FDA regulations of those facilities where drugs were being produced.

It was much simpler to just order what was commercially available and after all, those commercially prepared products had undergone FDA testing and approval before being brought to market availability. Though individual compounding of medications did not cease to exist, the demand for such products was drastically decreased.

Up until 1997, there were no formidable laws regarding the process of compounding in the pharmacy setting. However, federal legislation passed allowing pharmacists the right to compound medications on-site. This legislation, entitled the FDA Modernization Act of 1997, preserved the pharmacist-patient-practitioner relationship as the basis for the practice of compounding. The major provisions stated that compounded products made in the pharmacy setting did not need to follow the strict adherence to FDA approval as those in mass production settings.

Since traditionally compounded products are prepared to meet the needs of special patients and are not marketed to the general public, the safety and effectiveness as well as public health concerns are not as prominent. In most cases, the patients who use compounded products are those in pediatric, geriatric or special needs groups whose abilities to use medications differ from those of the typical adult patient. Sometimes a simple alteration of a commercially available product is all that is required. Other times, medications must be made from scratch with actual FDA approved active ingredients to meet a patient's need for medication.

A patient may simply need a different dose or dosage form in order to meet their needs, help them to adhere to a medication regimen or to reach therapeutic outcomes desired by their prescribers. There are many reasons why a patient might need the pharmacy to compound their medication.

Compounded Dosage Forms

Reconstitution of sterile products for parental use also involves adding approved compatible solvents to commercially available products according to manufacturer's instructions and does not constitute traditional compounding.

There are various forms of compounded products. Solutions are one of the most common forms of compounded products. A solution is a clear, but not necessarily colorless, liquid in which a drug in liquid or solid form has been dissolved. Two common types of solutions are syrups and elixirs. Syrups are commonly used for the liquid vehicle. Syrups are highly concentrated, almost saturated, mixtures of sucrose (sugar) and water. Elixirs are hydro-alcoholic solutions, meaning that they are made of alcohol and water. Elixirs are also often used for the liquid vehicle in a solution.

Another liquid form of compounded medications is a suspension. Many suspensions come pre-manufactured today in the form of powdered antibiotics ready for reconstitution. This type of suspension preparation does not fall within the ranks of traditional compounding. Reconstituting involves adding a compatible solvent such as sterile or distilled water to a product according to manufacturer's FDA approved instructions to achieve a specific concentration.

Still there are many needs for suspensions to be compounded in the pharmacy. Because of dosing needs and requirements, sometimes more ingredient than will dissolve into a reasonable amount of liquid is necessary. This makes the solution dosage form unacceptable for some medications and requires the compounding of a suspension.

Suspensions will be noticed as such because of their thick, sometimes almost creamy, texture. They consist of finely divided particles of a solid "powder" form of a medication dispersed evenly in a liquid vehicle. Since the particles will not fully dissolve, a suspending agent is generally used to "hold" the particles evenly dispersed until a dose can be administered. In a short time, the particles of a suspension will settle to the bottom of a container separating from the liquid vehicle in the product. Vigorous shaking will redistribute the particles evenly in the liquid so that an accurate dose of the medication can again be given to the patient.

A fortified strength would be stronger and a diluted strength would be weaker than what is commercially available.

Most suspensions compounded in the pharmacy will consist of: a liquid vehicle (water or syrup), a suspending agent that will thicken the liquid and a solid powder form of a medication. It might also be necessary to add a flavoring to the mixture to help mask the taste of the powdered medication.

Many physicians, especially dermatologists, will desire for their patient to have either a fortified strength or a diluted strength of medication than what is available from the manufacturer. For this reason, ointments and creams are also among the most requested forms of compounding. An ointment is an oil-based solid that is used for topical application. The texture of an ointment will be noticed by its greasiness. A cream is also used topically, but it is a water-based solid form that goes on more smoothly and is not greasy.

Emulsions are not as well heard of but they can also be compounded in the pharmacy. An emulsion consists of two immiscible liquids. One of the liquids will be dispersed throughout the other in the form of tiny droplets.

Many patients may need the pharmacy to compound their medication in the form of a suppository. Both rectal and vaginal suppositories can be very easily compounded with the right equipment. A semi-solid form of medication mixed with a base will be poured into suppository molds until they are set. Afterwards the reusable molds can be disassembled and removed. If the pharmacy chooses to use the disposable type there will be no need to remove the outer wrapping. What will remain will be a suppository that is ready for use by the patient.

Capsules can be prepared in the pharmacy setting. There are two main methods for such preparation. One method, known as the hand punch method, involves opening the empty shell of the capsule and filling it by hand, leveling off the excess and then capping off with the other end. The size of the chosen capsule shell would be based on the weight of medication it will accommodate.

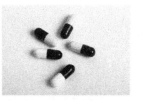

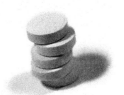

The other method involves the use of a capsule filling machine. Capsule shells would be separated into parts and placed in the empty machine. The weighed powdered filler (including active ingredient and any filler needed to make an appropriate weighted capsule) would be placed onto the machine bed. When turned on, the machine vibrates forcing the powder to fall into the empty half shells. The process continues until all the shells are filled appropriately and then the halves are capped off.

Empty gelatin shells that can be filled with medication come in a variety of sizes. Just as you learned with needle sizes, the larger the number, the smaller the size and vice versa also holds true with the empty capsule shells. 000 is the largest and 5 is the smallest. Sizes available are 000, 00, 0, 1, 2, 3, 4, and 5.

Tablets can be prepared with a special piece of equipment known as a tablet press. The press allows the powder substance to fall into a mold bed. When the machine is closed, it places enough pressure on the powdered substance to cause it to hold together and form a tablet. Tablets are not as commonly prepared in the pharmacy setting as are other dosage forms.

Compounding Equipment

Special equipment will be needed to practice compounding within a pharmacy. To measure, one would use equipment such as a balance, weights, weighing boats, graduates, pipettes, flasks, and syringes. In mixing, one could use beakers, flasks, spatulas, funnels, and mortar and pestles. Molding would necessitate the use of suppository molds, capsule shells or ointment slabs. After a medication is compounded, a prescription vial or bottle, ointment jar, or suppository box would be used to hold the medication for delivery to the patient.

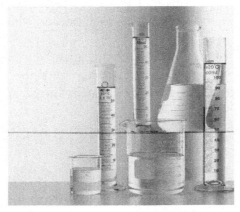

Balance and Weights

A prescription balance and a set of weights would be used in measuring just the right amount of a powdered or other solid medication to include in a compound. A torsion balance also referred to as the Class A prescription balance is just one type of balance. It is pictured below along with a weight set.

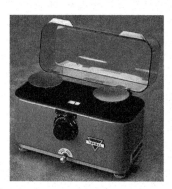 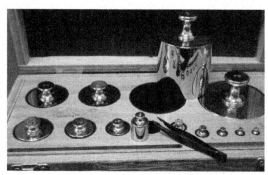

Proper Technique for Using a Class A Torsion Prescription Balance

*Move the balance from its storage location to the work counter.

*Level the balance first from front to back and then from side to side using the screw legs. The arrest knob will need to be unlocked during this adjustment so that the marker can freely move and will be visible when it is appropriately leveled back to the center. Arrest the balance.

*Place weighing boats or glassine papers onto each of the weighing pans, then unlock the balance and adjust the internal weight back to zero to allow for the variance in the weights of the two boats or papers.

*Using the tongs from the weight set; place the desired weight amount onto the weighing pan on the right. If a smaller amount of weight needs to be added, the large dial (the rider) can be turned to added increments of weight to the right weighing pan to coincide with the weight that has been already placed on there.

*Add the approximate weight of powdered substance to the boat on the left side weighing pan. Unlock the arrest knob to check the status of the weight. Lock it back each time an adjustment is made.

*When the desired weight is achieved, arrest the balance one final time. Remove the weighed substance, return the weights to their respective place and clean the balance with the appropriate cloth wipe.

A digital scale may also be used and is more popular today in specialty type pharmacies where substances are constantly being weighed. Pictured below are two additional scales.

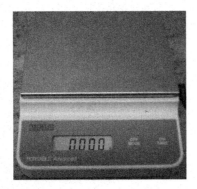 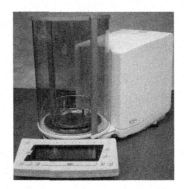

Liquid Measurement

When measuring liquids always use the smallest device that will accommodate the volume you are measuring for better accuracy. Use a volumetric container calibrated for delivery such as a graduate, syringe or pipette. Nonvolumetric devices such as beakers and prescription bottles are used to contain or hold medications after measurement and for use during the compounding are marked with approximate volumes. Accuracy should not be based on nonvolumetric container values. Notice that the graduated cylinder (pictured left), has markings that define each individually calibrated milliliter. The beaker on the right only has markings that begin with 400mL and are marked every 50mL up to 1000mL. The graduated cylinder is a volumetric container and the beaker is a nonvolumetric one.

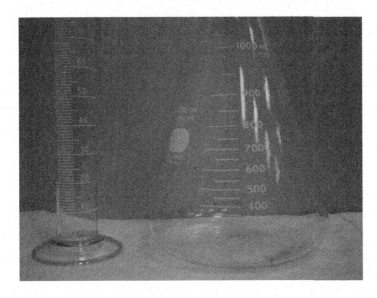 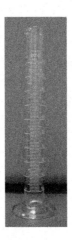

Any time liquids are measured there will be a meniscus. The narrower the diameter of the measuring device is, the more prominently visible the meniscus will be. This is the curved area at the surface of the liquid. It is formed because of the pressure of the liquid against the edge of the container. When reading the volume of liquid, hold the container so that the meniscus is at eye level and read the measurement from the bottom of the meniscus. The following diagram will give you better insight to explain what we mean. Compare it with the actual meniscus pictured below.

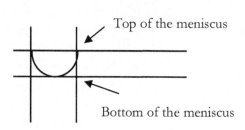

Top of the meniscus

Bottom of the meniscus

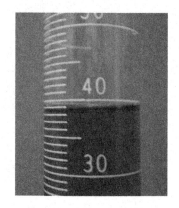

A mortar and pestle is a well-used piece of equipment in compounding pharmacy practice. In fact, it is probably the most iconic symbol in pharmacy history. The mortar is used to hold a medication while it is triturated or ground with the pestle. Depending upon what type of substance is being triturated would determine the type of mortar and pestle is best to use. For instance, powders and other solid surfaces are fine in most any type of set including ceramic, porcelain and other types. Liquids are best prepared in a glass set. The glass is non porous and resists stains better. Pictured below is a mortar and pestle set.

An ointment slab like the one pictured below will be used in levigation of ointments and creams. A spatula such as the one shown in the picture may be used to mix or levigate with until the mixture is homogenous or the same all the way through. Sometimes a handheld mixer called a homogenizer will be used to help with mixing and levigation of creams and lotions.

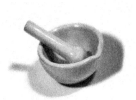

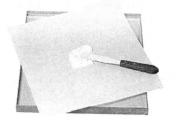

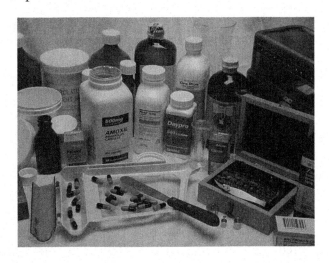

Math Blaster

The calculations used for compounding are some of the most difficult to learn because of the many steps involved. The mathematics used to calculate the weights and volumes needed for compounding go back to the simple adding, subtracting, multiplying and dividing. It is simply the matter of knowing how and where to put the numbers.

In this portion of the mission, the process of allegating between two strengths of a given substance to form a new strength will be learned. Figuring strengths, amounts and active ingredients for compounded products also is part of the upcoming lessons. Likewise, basic principles of working with concentrations and dilutions are studied also.

When working with the basics of pharmacy compounding, the units of these formulas will be measured in milliliters or grams which are the basic units of measurement. If other measurements are given or are needed afterwards, conversions must be performed.

Allegations

It is necessary to allegate when two different strengths or percents of a medication are mixed together to prepare a desired third strength. It can be determined how much of each strength will be needed based on the final amount, weight or volume that is being prepared. In order to allegate, one would need to have knowledge of three percent values.

First, the highest on hand or stock strength and second, the lowest on hand or stock strength are needed. Note there are times when a product is simply going to be diluted with water or petrolatum base that can be considered neutral or 0% as the lowest on hand or stock strength. Finally, a third percent strength or desired amount is presented as the product to be prepared and generally a specific weight or volume being compounded is also given.

Here is how the allegation chart should be set up.

Each block of the chart has a specific place and purpose as does each column (up and down) and row (across). Note the titles of each column below.

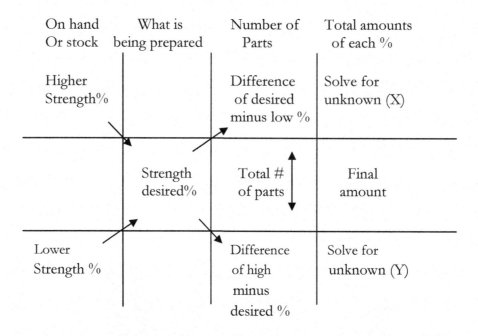

On hand Or stock	What is being prepared	Number of Parts	Total amounts of each %
Higher Strength%		Difference of desired minus low %	Solve for unknown (X)
	Strength desired%	Total # of parts	Final amount
Lower Strength %		Difference of high minus desired %	Solve for unknown (Y)

Here is a sample allegation problem:

You have of the same medication, a 9% ointment and 2% ointment. You get an order for 25gm of 5% ointment. How much of each strength will you need to make the 25gm of 5% ointment?

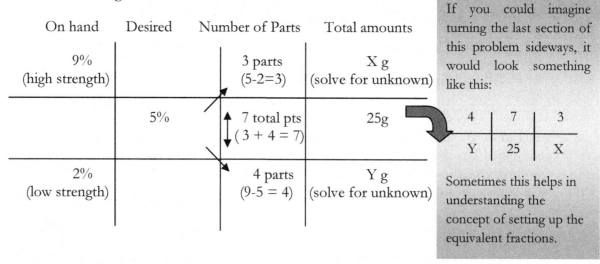

On hand	Desired	Number of Parts	Total amounts
9% (high strength)		3 parts (5-2=3)	X g (solve for unknown)
	5%	7 total pts (3 + 4 = 7)	25g
2% (low strength)		4 parts (9-5 = 4)	Y g (solve for unknown)

If you could imagine turning the last section of this problem sideways, it would look something like this:

4	7	3
Y	25	X

Sometimes this helps in understanding the concept of setting up the equivalent fractions.

$$\frac{4}{Y} = \frac{7}{25} \qquad\qquad \frac{7}{25} = \frac{3}{X} \qquad\qquad \text{Cross multiply to solve for unknowns}$$

$$4 \times 25 = 7 \times Y \qquad\qquad 7 \times X = 3 \times 25$$

$$100 = 7Y \qquad\qquad 7X = 75$$

$$\frac{}{7} \quad \frac{}{7} \qquad\qquad \frac{}{7} \quad \frac{}{7} \qquad\qquad \text{Divide by what's with the X and Ys.}$$

$$14.3g = Y \qquad\qquad X = 10.7g$$

Check yourself by adding the two amounts together to see if the sum equals the amount to be prepared. In this case, the 14.3g plus the 10.7g equals the 25g to be prepared.

10.7g of the 9% ointment and 14.3g of the 2% ointment will be needed to make 25g of the 5% ointment. Always be sure to keep the amounts and their percent strengths together. For instance, in the above calculation, X g is the measurement for the 9% and Y g is the measurement for the 2%. Each row is significant to it's percent strength. The 9% required 3 parts and totaled 10.7g. The 2% required 4 parts and totaled 14.3g. The product being compounded, 5%, required all 7 parts to prepare the 25g amount. Perhaps the color coded rows below will help explain this concept.

9%		3 parts	X = 10.7 g
	5%	7 total pts	25g
2%		4 parts	Y = 14.3g

Total Amount, Percent Strength and Active Ingredient

Determining the final percent strengths and the amounts of active ingredient in a compound should be commonplace with pharmacy technicians. In addition, if given this information (percent strength and amount of active ingredient) a technician should be able to calculate the total amount to be prepared.

There is one formula that can be used to perform all three calculations provided that two of the three figures are known. If you are asked to find the total amount, the final percentage strength or the active ingredient amount of a compounded mixture or liquid this formula will help you out.

$$TA \times \% = AI$$

The key thing to remember is that TA can represent the final volume or weight to be prepared and the AI represents the amount of active ingredient. The percent given can be used to multiply or divide with depending on which is the unknown portion of the compound. If looking for the final percent strength, the answer will first be given in decimal form. It must be converted to percent form. Multiplying the decimal by 100 can do this or you may simply move the decimal two places to the right. If necessary, review the lesson on decimals and percents in Mission 1.

.D P $\longrightarrow$ D P. $\longrightarrow$ %

.D P $\longleftarrow$ D P. $\longleftarrow$ %

Also, a percent may be given in the form of a ratio such as a 1:200. To use this figure in the above given formula you must also change the ratio to a percent form. If necessary, review the lesson on fractions, ratios, decimals and percents in Mission 2.

1:200 $\longrightarrow$ $\dfrac{1}{200}$

becomes

$1 \div 200 = 0.005$

0.005 becomes 0.5%

When learning to perform these calculations, there is a helping hint for learning to set the problems up. The word "of" can be replaced by a multiplication (x) sign. The words will deliver, is, that contains and to make can all be replaced with the equals (=) sign.

Let's work through some examples.

You have ciprofloxacin 5% oral suspension. How many grams of active ingredient are in 125mL of suspension?

$$
\begin{array}{rlll}
TA & x & \% & = & AI \\
125mL & x & 5\% & = & AI \\
& & 6.25g & = & AI
\end{array}
$$

There are 6.25 grams of active ingredient in ciprofloxacin 5% oral suspension.

How many grams of 20% zinc oxide ointment will deliver 8 g of zinc oxide?

$$TA \times \% = AI$$
$$TA \times 20\% = 8g$$
$$20\%TA = 8$$

$$\frac{20\%}{} \qquad \frac{20\%}{}$$

$$TA = 40$$

40g of zinc oxide ointment will deliver 8g of zinc oxide.

_____

A technician in the pharmacy has compounded 50g silver nitrate ointment that contains 1 gram of silver nitrate. What percentage strength should the ointment be labeled?

$$TA \times \% = AI$$
$$50g \times X = 1g$$
$$50X = 1$$

$$\frac{50}{} \qquad \frac{50}{}$$

$$X = 0.02 \text{ or } 2\% \quad \text{(Don't forget to convert to percent form)}$$

The ointment should be labeled as 2% silver nitrate ointment.

Concentrations and Dilutions

Concentrations and dilutions are routinely used in the compounding pharmacy. A technician should be knowledgeable of the procedure to perform these calculations. At times, you may have in stock a concentrated or pure form of a certain solution. When a doctor orders a specific concentration (percent strength) of that solution, the stock solution must be diluted to that specific concentration.

Calculate the total amount or concentration based on the initial figures for amounts and percentage strengths. Sometimes the initial volume or percentage strength will be calculated based on given figures for final amounts and strengths. There are four place values to the formula used to perform these calculations. As long as three of the four values are known, the unknown one can be determined.

$$A_1\ P_1 = A_2\ P_2$$

To understand this formula, A_1 equals the amount of the first (initial) solution or compound. P_1 equals the percent strength or concentration of the first (initial) solution or compound. The A_2 represents the amount of the second (final) solution or compound. P_2 equals the percent strength or concentration of the second (final) solution or compound.

The key idea is to make sure to keep the correct amounts and percentages together that go together. Any of the four areas of the calculation can be found providing that the other 3 figures are given. As in the formula before, the answers will be given in milliliters or grams and follow up conversions may have to be performed to finish the problem. Here are some sample questions:

If 500ml of a 15% solution are diluted to 1500ml, what will the final percent strength be?

$$
\begin{array}{ccccc}
A_1 & x & P_1 & = & A_2 & x & P_2 \\
\end{array}
$$

500mL x 15% = 1500mL x X%

75 = 1500X

$$\frac{75}{1500} \quad \frac{1500X}{1500}$$

0.05 or 5% = X

(Don't forget to convert answer to percent form.)

The final solution of 1500ml will be a 5% solution.

Think logically to check your answer initially. The volume or amount of the compound will increase and the percent strength will decrease with this process. This will happen proportionally. For instance, the volume here started out as 500mL and increased to 1500mL which is three times the amount of the original solution. On the contrary, the strength started out a 15% and was reduced to 5% which is one-third of the original strength.

The A's are amounts and may be either grams or milliliters.

The P's are percents. If a strength in another form such as a decimal or ratio is given, it must be converted.

The 1's represent the initial or starting amounts and percents.

The 2's represent the final or ending amounts and percents.

What volume of 5% aluminum acetate solution will be needed to make 120ml of a 0.05% solution?

$$A_1 \quad x \quad P_1 \quad = \quad A_2 \quad x \quad P_2$$
$$X \quad x \quad 5\% \quad = \quad 120mL \quad x \quad 0.05\%$$
$$5\%X \quad = \quad 0.06$$

$$\frac{5\%}{5\%} \quad \frac{5\%}{}$$

$$X \quad = \quad 1.2$$

1.2ml of the 5% solution will be needed to compound the 120ml of 0.05% solution.

Again, the volume or amount of the compound will increase and the percent strength will decrease proportionally. Here the volume here started out as 1.2mL and increased to 120mL which is one hundred times the amount of the original solution. On the contrary, the strength started out a 5% and was reduced to 0.05% which is one-hundredth of the original strength.

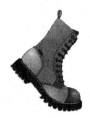

Drill Practice

Complete the following calculations then check yourself in the rear of the textbook. Sometimes a problem may require several steps to solve.

Allegate the following.

1. An order for 1 lb 4% zinc oxide paste is prepared using the pharmacy's stock 10% paste and 1% paste. How much of each stock paste must be mixed to obtain the desired concentration? [Assume 1 lb = 454 g]

2. To process a prescription order for a 12.5% dextrose solution, the pharmacy technician would mix the stock solutions of 20% dextrose and 5% dextrose solutions to make 1L of the 12.5% solution? How much of each strength stock solution will be needed?

3. The povidone iodine solution your pharmacy stocks is 10%. A patient brings a script for 3% povidone iodine solution, 12 oz to use as directed. How much 10% stock solution and water will you need to compound this mixture? [hint: water is 0%]

4. The pharmacy has a 10% strength and a 2% strength of the same ointment. An order comes in for 8oz of 5% ointment. How much 2% ointment would be needed?

5. To process a prescription order for a 4% solution, the pharmacy technician would mix the stock solutions of 6% solution and water. How much of each would be needed to make a pint (480ml) of the 4 % solution?

Determine the appropriate total amount, strength or active ingredient.

6. Determine the amount of 1.5% hydrocortisone cream that can be prepared from 1.8g of hydrocortisone powder mixed into a cream base.

7. How much gentian violet is in 120 mL of a 1:10,000 solution?

8. How should the final product be labeled if 200mL of metronidazole suspension contains 4.8 grams of active ingredient?

9. How much neomycin powder must be added to fluocinolone cream to dispense an order for 60 g of fluocinolone cream with 0.5% neomycin?

10. How many grams of 2% silver nitrate ointment will deliver 5g of the active ingredient?

11. The stock ciprofloxacin oral suspension contains 5 grams of active ingredient in 125ml of suspension?

Solve the following concentrations and dilutions.

12. You have 20ml of a 1:200 solution in stock. If the pharmacist has asked you to dilute the solution to 500ml, how would you label the final strength?

13. If 300ml of a 15% solution are diluted to 1200ml, what will the final percent strength be?

14. What volume of 6% solution will be needed to make 120ml of a 0.3% solution?

15. 50ml of a 1:10 solution in stock. If the pharmacist has asked you to dilute the solution to 2.5%, how many milliliters can be prepared?

Solve the following compounding problems.

16. To prepare an order for 25g of 1.5% hydrocortisone ointment, how much of 2.5% and 1% hydrocortisone ointments will be needed?

17. If 2oz of ibuprofen ointment contains 12g of ibuprofen, with what strength should the package be labeled?

18. If the technician has prepared a 450g jar of sugardine ointment for use in the wound care center, how many grams of 10% povidone iodine ointment were included if the final strength is labeled at 4%?

19. You've been asked to prepare 4% Trolamine lotion using the stock 10% cream and diluting it with hydrophor base. How much of each will you need to make the 4oz the physician has ordered for the patient?

20. Acetic acid otic solution has been ordered for a patient. Using 22.5mL of the pharmacy's stock 4% solution to compound the 60mL ordered amount, how will you label the final strength of the prescription?

Drug Training Chapter Six

Brand Name	Generic Name	Drug Classification	Primary Indication	Side effects, Warnings, Other
Neurontin	Gabapentin	Anti-Convulsant	postherpetic neuralgia and adjunctive therapy for seizures	dizziness, somnolence, and peripheral edema
Wellbutrin XL	Bupropion	Anti-Depressant (Aminoketone class)	Major Depressive Disorder	May increase risk of suicidal thinking and behavior in children, adolescents, and young adults; May also cause agitation, dry mouth, insomnia, headache/migraine, nausea/vomiting, constipation, and tremor.
Glucophage	Metformin	Anti-Hyperglycemic	Type 2 Diabetes	Abnormal stools, hypoglycemia, myalgia, lightheaded, dyspnea, flushing, palpitation
Elavil	Amitriptyline	Tricyclic Anti-Depressant	Depression	Cardiac arrythmias, orthostatic hypotension, ataxia, parasthesia, rash
Imitrex	Sumatriptan	Serotonin Receptor Agonist	Acute treatment of migraine headaches	Serious cardiac events have occurred post use; may also cause parasthesia, atypical sensations and pain in various areas
Cialis	Tadalafil	ED agent	Erectile Dysfunction	Headache, dyspepsia, flushing, pain in extremities
Crestor	Rosuvastatin	Lipid-Lowering Agent	Hyperlipidemia, Dyslipidemia	May increase risk of Rhabdomyolysis, acute renal failure, myopathy, liver enzyme abnormalities; may also cause headache, abdominal pain and/or nausea, myalgia, asthenia

Brand Name	Generic Name	Drug Classification	Primary Indication	Side effects, Warnings, Other
Geodon	ziprasidone	antispsychotic	schizophrenia, bipolar disorder	Elderly patients with dementia-related psychosis treated with antipsychotic drugs are at an increased risk of death
Actos	Pioglitazone	Thiazolidinediones	Type 2 Diabetes	May cause or exacerbate CHF, also may increase risk of URI
Lotrisone	Clotrimazole/ Betamethasone	Topical Antifungal Corticosteroid Combination	treatment of symptomatic inflammatory tinea pedis, tinea cruris, and tinea corporis	Parasthesia, rash, edema and secondary infection
Aciphex	Rabeprazole	Proton Pump Inhibitor	Gastroesophageal Reflux Disease (GERD), duodenal ulcers	Headache, Abdominal Pain, Dry Mouth, Dizziness
Deltasone	Prednisone	Glucocorticoid	Various uses including allergic treatments, GI disorders, respiratory and arthritic conditions and more.	Cardiac arrythmias, vertigo, headache, paresthesia, development of cushingoid state (ie moonface, buffalo hump) fluid retention, weight gain and others

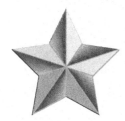

Mission 6 Debriefing

Answer the following questions in assessment of the lessons learned in Mission 6. For best results, repeat the exercise until no questions are missed then move on to the next mission.

1. Which of the following pairs of medications are indicated for type 2 diabetes?
   a) gabapentin and rosuvastatin
   b) metformin and bupropion
   c) gabapentin and pioglitazone
   d) pioglitazone and metformin

2. Creams are oil-based topical that absorb smoothly and are not greasy.
   a) True
   b) False

3. After moving the class A torsion prescription balance to the work counter, the next step is to
   _____.
   a) Place the weighing boats or glassine papers onto the pans
   b) Use the tongs and add the weights from the weight set
   c) Level the balance using the screw legs.
   d) Add the substance to be weighed to the pan on the right.

4. Some probable candidates for using or requiring compounded products are _____.
   a) pediatrics
   b) geriatrics
   c) special needs patients
   d) all of these

5. Fortifying a compounded product makes it _____ than the original product.
   a) weaker
   b) stronger

6. Prior to 1950 about _____ of medications were compounded in the pharmacy setting.
   a) 20%
   b) 50%
   c) 60%
   d) 80%

7. Containers such as _____ and _____ should not be used to accurately measure desired volumes.
   a) beakers and prescription bottles
   b) graduates or syringes
   c) pipettes and graduates
   d) pipettes and syringes

8. Adding the weights from the weight set to the prescription balance should be done with the tongs and not by a bare hand.
   a) True
   b) False

9. The sensitivity of a Class A torsion prescription balance is _____.
   a) 6mg
   c) 6g
   b) 120mg
   d) There is no measurable sensitivity

10. A solution is a clear but not necessarily colorless liquid in which a substance has been completely dissolved.
   a) True
   b) False

11. The FDA Modernization Act was passed in what year?
   a) 1951
   c) 1990
   b) 1970
   d) 1997

12. Tadalafil is primarily indicated for _____.
   a) erectile dysfunction
   c) GERD
   b) diabetes
   d) Hyperlipidemia

13. _____ are helpful when the dosing needs or requirements will not dissolve completely into a reasonable amount of liquid.
   a) Solutions
   c) Suspensions
   b) Elixers
   d) Syrups

14. Which of the following is a topically applied compound dosage form?
   a) Cream
   c) Both a and b
   b) Ointment
   d) Neither a nor b

15. A patient has been diagnosed with GERD. Which of the following medications is likely to be prescribed?
   a) Actos
   c) Glucophage
   b) Aciphex
   d) Crestor

16. A _____ is used in measuring liquids for preparing compounded dosage forms.
   a) spatula
   c) graduate
   b) mortar
   d) beaker

17. Weighing boats or glassine papers should be added to which pan(s) on the weighing balance?
   a) Right
   c) Both
   b) Left
   d) only where the powder is

18. Solutions are commonly compounded in the pharmacy setting. Which of the following are solutions?
   a) Elixers
   c) Both a and b
   b) Syrups
   d) Neither a nor b

19. Prednisone is a glucocorticoid agent.
   a) True
   b) False

20. When adding the solid or powdered substance to be weighed onto a Class A torsion prescription balance, it should be placed into the pan on the _____.
   a) right
   b) left
   c) either side

21. Which decade brought the "birth" of mass manufactured medications and FDA regulations of those facilities?
   a) 1940's
   b) 1950's
   c) 1960's
   d) 1980's

22. Which of the following would not be used in "mixing" a compounded product?
   a) Pipette
   b) Syringe
   c) Beaker
   d) Weighing boat

23. Compounded products made in the pharmacy setting are not marketed to the general public but are primarily for those whose abilities to use traditional medications differ from the typical patient.
   a) True
   b) False

24. Which of the following is a topical steroid/antifungal combination?
   a) Deltasone
   b) Lotrisone
   c) Crestor
   d) Neurontin

25. Dilution of a compound makes it _____ than the original product.
   a) weaker
   b) stronger

26. Making _____ requires the use of pouring molds.
   a) creams
   b) suppositories
   c) lotions
   d) elixers

27. Geodon is used in treating _____.
   a) inflammation
   b) depression
   c) schizophrenia
   d) hyperlipidemia

28. When measuring liquids always use the largest device on hand to make sure that it will accommodate the volume of liquid to be measured.
   a) True
   b) False

29. When adding weights to the Class A prescription balance, they should be placed in the pan on the _____.
   a) right
   b) left

30. Mixing manufacturer prepared antibiotic suspensions constitutes another form of traditional compounding.
   a) True
   b) False

31. Elderly patients with dementia related psychosis treated with antipsychotic drugs are at an increased risk of death.
   a) True
   b) False

32. The _____ is used to "hold" the substance while it is triturated with the _____.
    a) ointment slab, spatula
    b) graduate, funnel
    c) mortar, pestle
    d) mold, spatula

33. Using steroids such as prednisone can cause such side effects as weight gain, fluid retention and development of cushingoid state such as moonface and/or buffalo hump.
    a) True
    b) False

34. Two immiscible liquids that are mixed together as a compounded dosage form become a(n)_____.
    a) cream
    b) syrup
    c) ointment
    d) emulsion

35. Which of the following pairs of medications are indicated for depression?
    a) Neurontin and Glucophage
    b) Wellbutrin XL and Elavil
    c) Cialis and Glucophage
    d) Crestor and Deltasone

36. A press is used in preparing tablet dosage forms in the pharmacy setting.
    a) True
    b) False

37. Neurontin is actually classed as a(n) _____ though it has many uses.
    a) anticonvulsant
    b) antihyperglycemic
    c) antihyperlipidemic
    d) ED agent

38. A pipette is a nonvolumetric measuring device.
    a) True
    b) False

39. A size _____ capsule is the smallest available empty gelatin shell for compounding.
    a) 00
    b) 5
    c) 0
    d) 1

40. While adding the substance to be weighed onto the balance, the arrest knob should be _____.
    a) locked
    b) unlocked

41. Which of the following compounded substances is a highly concentrated mixture of sucrose and water?
    a) Solution
    b) Suspension
    c) Syrup
    d) Elixir

42. A tablet press uses _____ to form tablets during the compounding process.
    a) heat
    b) pressure
    c) both a and b
    d) neither a nor b

43. Sumatriptan is indicated to treat major depressive disorder
    a) True
    b) False

44. A _____ and _____ could be used in measuring just the right amount of a powdered or solid medication to include in a compound.
   a) ointment slab and spatula
   c) prescription balance and weights
   b) mortar and pestle
   d) tray and spatula

45. Tablets and emulsions are some of the most commonly compounded products in the pharmacy setting.
   a) True
   b) False

46. Which of the following is likely to be included in the preparation of a compounded suspension.
   a) Liquid vehicle such as water or a syrup
   b) A suspending agent for thickening and distribution of particles
   c) Solid powder form of a medication
   d) All of these

47. If disposable suppository molds are used there is no need to open them after preparation.
   a) True
   b) False

48. Liquids are best mixed in a _____ mortar and pestle set because they are non-porous and resist stains.
   a) Glass
   c) Ceramic
   b) Porcelain
   d) Wood

49. We may compound in the pharmacy setting to _____.
   a) provide a different dosage form that what is commercially available.
   b) help a patient adhere to a medication regimen.
   c) help a patient reach their prescriber's desired therapeutic outcomes.
   d) any and all of these.

50. If a substance is homogenous, it is the same consistency all the way through the entire product.
   a) True
   b) False

51. A patient's recent labwork shows she has high cholesterol levels. Which of these medications might be prescribed for her as a result?
   a) Imitrex
   c) Glucophage
   b) Geodon
   d) Crestor

52. What should be done as a final step of using the Class A torsion prescription balance before returning it to the proper storage area?
   a) The weights should be returned to their respective place.
   b) The balance should be wiped with an appropriate cloth wipe.
   c) The weighing boats or papers should be discarded.
   d) None of these.

53. Which of the following drugs may cause a risk of suicidal thoughts in children, adolescents and young adults?
   a) Wellbutrin XL
   c) Crestor
   b) Cialis
   d) Geodon

54. A handheld mixer called a(n) _____ is sometimes used in the mixing of creams, ointments and other semi-solid preparations such as creams, ointments and lotions.
   a) Oxidizer
   b) Shaker
   c) Mortar
   d) Homogenizer

55. Suspensions require vigorous shaking to redistribute particles that have settled so that an accurate dose can be given each and every time.
   a) True
   b) False

56. A(n) _____ is an oil-based dosage form with a very greasy texture.
   a) Ointment
   b) Cream
   c) Emulsion
   d) Lotion

57. A graduate is a nonvolumetric container.
   a) True
   b) False

58. Rosuvastatin tends to cause an increase in the risk of _____.
   a) Suicidal thinking in children, adolescents and young adults
   b) Abnormal liver enzymes
   c) Death in elderly patients
   d) Abnormal stools

59. Which of these could be used to hold medications for patient delivery and use?
   a) Prescription vials and bottles
   b) Suppository box
   c) Ointment jar
   d) Any of these could be used

60. An elixir is hydroalcoholic.
   a) True
   b) False

61. The FDA Modernization Act of 1997 offered provisions for compounding in the pharmacy setting without strict adherence to requirements for compounding in mass production settings.
   a) True
   b) False

62. It is necessary to _____ when two different strengths, one higher and one lower, of a medication or substance are mixed together to prepare a desired third "in-between" strength.
   a) Dilute
   b) Fortify
   c) Allegate
   d) None of these

63. Reconstituting a manufacturer's prepared unit such as an injectable or oral antibiotic with sterile or distilled water according to accompanied directions will achieve a specified concentration if mixed correctly and therefore does not constitute traditional compounding.
   a) True
   b) False

64. Which of the following methods for preparing capsule dosage forms includes filling one end of an empty gelatin shell and leveling off the excess before capping off with the other end of the gelatin shell?
   a) The hand punch method
   b) Using a capsule filling machine
   c) Either a or b
   d) Neither a nor b

65. A meniscus is curved area formed at the surface of a liquid and should be read from the _____.
   a) Top
   b) Middle
   c) Bottom
   d) Neither of these

66. An ointment slab and spatula is used in _____ of ointments and other topical preparations.
   a) trituration
   b) levigation
   c) allegation
   d) saturation

67. A _____ is thick and creamy like and consists of finely divided particles dispersed evenly in a liquid vehicle.
   a) solution
   b) elixir
   c) emulsion
   d) suspension

68. Using the large knob on the Class A torsion prescription balance, a small amount of additional weight can be added to coincide with the already added weight on the _____ pan.
   a) right
   b) left

69. Which is the largest empty gelatin shell size used in compounding capsules in the pharmacy setting?
   a) 5
   b) 0
   c) 00
   d) 000

70. The minimum accurate weight that can be measured on a Class A torsion prescription balance is _____.
   a) 6mg
   b) 120mg
   c) 120g
   d) There is no minimum weight

Number the statements 71-76 below in the order they should go when using a Class A torsion prescription balance. For instance, the first step should get number 1, the next step, number 2 and so on. Please note that the technique is not included in entirety but each step can appropriately be numbered as instructed.

71. _____ Remove the weighed substance, return the weights to their proper place and clean the balance.
72. _____ Using correct technique, add the desired amount of weight to the appropriate pan.
73. _____ Move the balance from the storage location to the work counter.
74. _____ Add the approximate amount of substance to be weighed to the appropriate pan.
75. _____ Level the balance using the screw legs.
76. _____ Place weighing boats or glassine papers on the balance.

154

Match the following drugs to their generic names.

77. Geodon   _____ a) gabapentin

78. Crestor   _____ b) tadalafil

79. Neurontin   _____ c) pioglitazone

80. Deltasone   _____ d) prednisone

81. Elavil   _____ e) ziprasidone

82. Actos   _____ f) bupropion

83. Imitrex   _____ g) metformin

84. Aciphex   _____ h) clotrimazole/betamethasone

85. Wellbutrin XL   _____ i) rabeprazole

86. Cialis   _____ j) amitriptyline

87. Glucophage   _____ k) sumatriptan

88. Lotrisone   _____ l) rosuvastatin

Match the following drugs to their classifications.

89. Gabapentin   _____ a) glucocorticoid

90. Metformin   _____ b) proton pump inhibitor

91. Sumatriptan   _____ c) topical antifungal/steroid

92. Rosuvastatin   _____ d) thiazolidinedione

93. Pioglitazone   _____ e) antipsychotic agent

94. Rabeprazole   _____ f) ED agent

95. Prednisone   _____ g) lipid lowering agent

96. Bupropion   _____ h) serotonin receptor agonist

97. Amitriptyline   _____ i) tricyclic antidepressant

98. Tadalafil   _____ j) antihyperglycemic agent

99. Clotrimazole/betamethasone   _____ k) aminoketone antidepressant

100. Ziprasidone   _____ l) anticonvulsant

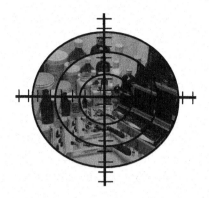

Mission 7
Purchasing, Procurement and Inventory Management

Mission Objectives

*To understand procedures necessary in ordering, receiving and storing pharmaceuticals.

*To identify proper storage requirements and conditions for pharmaceuticals.

*To recognize the purpose for MSDS sheets and correct handling of hazardous substances.

*To identify the various parts and purposes of a National Drug Code number.

*To understand the processes by which items are removed from inventory.

*To become knowledgeable of procedures for repackaging bulk pharmaceuticals.

*To recognize and implement procedures for reducing medication errors.

*To recognize the most common automated dispensing systems.

*Maintain records, routine inventories and area inspections.

*To gain baseline knowledge of twelve of the most popular drugs on the market.

*To understand the principles of pharmacy business calculations.

Managing the pharmacy's inventory is typically assigned to a specific person or small team of individuals. However, in actuality, proper inventory management requires effort from the entire pharmacy team. Most often it is a pharmacy technician that is assigned the position of inventory manager and the task is a job that can be handled well by a skillful technician. With that being said, the inventory manager will depend on daily support from the entire pharmacy staff to be a successful in the position.

Your pharmacy will probably follow an established procedure for purchasing and management of inventory. The guidelines for the proper procedures for this task could be found in the pharmacy's Policy and Procedures Manual. This is especially true if the pharmacy is within a healthcare setting such as a hospital or within a chain pharmacy system. Independent store owners may not have per say, this type of manual. Instead, the privately owned pharmacy may be operated on an unwritten but yet "understood by all" type set of rules.

Maintaining the inventory for pharmacy services can be quite the challenge for all involved. For the most part, the normal day to day operations of this position are routine and infallible. However, it's those days when things don't go as planned, that an inventory manager is put to the test. If a pharmacy doesn't have what is needed when it is needed, then the patients are the ones who must go lacking and therefore suffer the most.

Purchasing Systems and Vendors

There are several different types of purchasing systems. Ordering direct from each of the individual manufacturers may result in a significant cost savings for the pharmacy. However, that savings comes at a price of inconvenience. There are so many different manufacturers putting pharmaceuticals on the market that to order from each one would be quite the hassle. Accounts would have to be set up with each individual company and payments and shipping would result between the pharmacy and each of the individual "vendors". This would be very time consuming and inconvenient for day to day maintenance of inventory.

Group purchasing organizations or wholesalers are more popular than direct purchasing for pharmacies in today's world. In this type system, the savings or "contract pricing" is balanced on the dollar value of the regular purchases from that wholesaler or organization. Therefore, the more money that is spent, the better contract pricing agreements between wholesaler and pharmacy will be. This is especially true when large chains or groups (i.e. the Department of Defense – which includes all military bases, VA hospitals, Public Health Service facilities and more) are purchasing under the same contract.

Purchasing may include several different suppliers or vendors. One supplier might be specifically for purchasing pharmaceuticals, while another supplier may sell equipment and supplies. Moreover, other suppliers may supply the pharmacy with yet another array of items. A contract with a primary wholesaler or prime vendor in which the pharmacy generally agrees to purchase 80-90% of their pharmaceutical needs from that wholesaler is known as a prime vendor agreement. This does not mean that items cannot be purchased from another source. All other vendors will be known as secondary vendors.

Purchasing Documents

There are two documents that can be used to track a purchase. To start, a purchase order is initiated when the order is being prepared for submission to the vendor. Purchase orders, also known as POs, are used to track those items that have been ordered until they are received. An invoice, on the other hand, is initiated from the wholesaler's end when they prepare the order for shipment. Once the pharmacy receives the order, each item is compared line by line
with the listed items on the invoice. Therefore, the invoice is also a type of document that is used to track purchases.

Another document that technicians deal with on a regular basis is a packing slip. When an order of any kind is received, it should contain either an invoice or a packing slip. A packing slip will most likely be attached to the box, tote or other type of container. Though technically, the packing slip cannot be used to track a purchase, it will show the quantities ordered and packaged in each shipment. This packing slip is not a bill, but it can be kept for records to compare with the invoice and/or statements from that vendor. If the invoice isn't included with the packing slip or shipment, it will probably be mailed to the pharmacy separately. A monthly statement will likely be mailed in addition to the invoice.

General Ordering Procedures

Most all pharmaceuticals can be ordered without any special documentation required. These regular items include OTC items, legend drugs, and controlled drugs in scheduled classes III, IV and V. Class II scheduled drugs require a bit more effort to acquire and the process for doing so will be discussed later on in the mission.

In recent years, the majority of wholesale ordering has become possible to do over the Internet. Most primary wholesalers and even secondary vendors will likely have an online catalog for use in ordering. This is helpful when looking for a particular item, item number, or price because items within the online catalog can usually be sorted in a manner of the inventory manager's choosing with a simple click. Even though, most pharmacies are ordering electronically, it's possible that some pharmacies are still using a handheld telxon to send a daily order. Even if a pharmacy does use a computer generated order system, an old fashioned "want book" is helpful to have on hand. This want book is a simple list of things that need to be placed on the order at the end of the day.

In the age of our current technologies, most pharmacies are on a "point" system where inventory management is concerned. In this type system, stock is inventoried and controlled via the computer. As prescriptions are filled, inventory is automatically decreased. Likewise, when an order is received, the inventory is automatically increased. When inventory on a item is set at a certain ordering point and the stock level drops below that set amount, the computer generated order system places that such item on an order list. When the order is placed, a predetermined order amount is requested. (For instance, 2 bottles)

This order will be transmitted to the wholesaler via Internet or modem at the close of business day or by a set deadline or cutoff ordering time established by the wholesaler. Most major wholesalers offer next day delivery every day of the week except Sundays. Many pharmacies only order during the weekdays Monday through Friday.

When the order is delivered, the inventory manager or other assigned pharmacy staff will be responsible for receiving it and checking it in according to the policy and procedures manual for the pharmacy. This should be done in an area away from the main flow of traffic to deter theft; especially, if there are controlled substances involved. As the order is checked in, a line-by-line comparison of the included invoice or packing slip should be done. As the items are put away into stock, the stock should be stored so that the earliest expiration dates are toward the shelf front, so that the earlier dated items can be used first. This process of placing items on the shelf is called stock rotation.

As pharmaceutical products are placed on the shelf, take note to glance at the expiration date. Occasionally, something will be received from the wholesaler that is already expired or very short-dated. The wholesaler should be notified of any expired, damaged or shorted items.

Storage patterns vary from pharmacy to pharmacy. Some facilities store pharmaceuticals in Alpha-Brand order. This means that items are stored in their particular segregated areas alphabetically by the brand name. For instance, the drug atenolol is generic for the brand name product of Tenormin. Therefore, atenolol would be placed in the "T" section where Tenormin would be located if it was a stocked item.

Other pharmacies choose to use an Alpha-Generic storage system whereby all items are stored in the proper area alphabetically by their generic names. In this case, atenolol would be stored in the "A" section and so would its brand name version of Tenormin because of the storage by generic name. There are some retailers that choose to use the alphabetical approach for all items, which would place the atenolol generic product in the As and the Tenormin brand product in the Ts.

Where controlled substances are concerned, the CIIs are generally under additional lock and key in a storage cabinet, vault or safe. CIII, IV and Vs may be stored under the conditions above by either brand or generic name. However, some pharmacies choose because of the controlled status of these medications to place them under additional lock and key also. As long as the controlled substances are not left out on the shelf in a specific "marked" area for controlled substances, they are fine on the shelf and this is the more commonly used procedure for storing controlled substances.

Generally there are pricing stickers for the OTC merchandise and for the pharmaceuticals. As items are pulled from the order tote or bin, they are "stickered" and prepared to be place into inventory. The pricing sticker should never cover pertinent information such as drug name, strength, lot number, expiration date or bar code.

Sometimes these pricing stickers are written in a special code. This will usually include the date of receipt, AWP (Average Wholesale Price) and net cost. Typically, the invoice number is also included on the sticker; however, it all depends on how the pharmacy requested the stickers to be set up when the account was opened. If pricing codes are used, something

similar to the example below will likely be followed. A pricing code would probably consist of a ten-letter word or phrase with no duplicate letters. An example would be:

P I N K F L O W E R
1 2 3 4 5 6 7 8 9 0

Jones RX
06B2
6831280
EOFN
LKWI

The date would be written 13A2, which would mean that this was received on the 13th of January 2012. The months are symbolized by the alphabet...A for January, B for February, and C for March and so on. The last digit of the year number will be included. At left is an example of a pricing sticker.

The invoice number would be present, as well. The AWP is normally located above the net cost. These would likely be written in "code" that would need to be deciphered by the pharmacy's pricing code such as the example above. In this case, the AWP of EOFN represents 9753 or $97.53, whereas the net cost of the item LKWI represents 6482 or $64.82. Using code helps to include more information without a lot of space. This information can play a key role in inventory control as it allows the pharmacy to monitor the turnover rate among other things.

Special Ordering Procedures for Scheduled II Drugs

Since Class II scheduled drug have the most potential for abuse, they are also the most difficult to acquisition. They can be procured in one of two ways. The manual order requires a special document for DEA purposes and stands as the order for the CIIs. It must be mailed or hand delivered to the wholesaler. It cannot be transmitted via fax, Internet or modem or telephone with a telxon machine. The other way is an electronic submission of the order via CSOS otherwise known as the Controlled Substances Ordering System.

The DEA document 222C is a triplicate copy document. After the 222C form has been completed, the pharmacy keeps copy 3, which is the back "blue" copy. Once the order has been received by the wholesaler and processed, the wholesaler keeps the original white copy 1. After the order has been filled and shipped by the wholesaler, the DEA office gets copy 2, which is the middle "green" copy, forwarded to them from the wholesaler.

This document must not have any over markings or errors or the wholesaler will reject it. If any errors are made, the form must be voided and kept on file in the pharmacy. The forms must all be accounted for and when more are needed, upon request, the DEA will mail them direct to the pharmacy.

As for the alternative method of procurement for these Class II drugs, the DEA now allows ordering through the CSOS, Controlled Substances Ordering System. This effort by the DEA has helped to solve many a dilemma revolving around the need for schedule II drugs. The process is made possible and remains equally secure through the acquirement of both a digital certificate and a digital signature. Technicians are not eligible staff to receive or request this digital signature or certificate though. The responsibility falls on the pharmacists.

Once an order is placed online through the wholesaler as any other order would be processed, the system realizes that the order contains requests for CIIs. At that point, the digital certificate is attached to the order and the submitting pharmacist is prompted to enter his/her digital signature for secure ordering. An electronic "match" must occur with the digital certificate and the digital signature in order for the requested purchase order to be accepted by the wholesaler. If all is well, the order is usually delivered next day along with the rest of the day's ordered items.

Anytime new advancements in technology arise, there are implementation costs, advantages and yes, disadvantages. For this reason, the newer CSOS opportunity is now an option but not a requirement for pharmacies. Business as usual continues for those who choose not to seek the digital certificates and signatures to take advantage of online submission for CIIs. Compare below the manual paper form DEA222C forms versus the newer electronic version through CSOS.

Manual DEA222C	CSOS
Ordering errors are frequent	Errors less frequent
Limited line items on a single PO	Unlimited line items on a single PO
Turnaround time about 3 days minimum	Next day delivery
Less frequent orders result in more stockpiling	More frequent ordering means less stockpiling
May require waiting for new forms	No preprinted forms needed.

When controlled substances are concerned, whether they are II's, III's, IV's or V's, the invoice is proof of receipt. The personnel responsible for purchasing will normally sign the invoice when the controlled substances are received. The technician should also have a countersignature by a pharmacist on duty to verify that the controlled substances were received.

There should be three different files for invoices based on the control status of the different medications. The different files are: Class II controlled substances, Classes III, IV and V controlled substances and those items which are non-controlled legend drugs and over-the-counter items. In the event of an audit by a third party payer such as Medicaid or other contracted insurance, yielding of any and all invoices and other documents is necessary and required.

Stock Outs, Back Orders and Drop Shipments

Normally, items will be in stock and awaiting order at your wholesaler. In the case of a temporarily out of stock, this just simply means that the wholesaler is awaiting a shipment from the manufacturer with the expected arrival date within a few days. When an item goes on manufacturer's back order, which means that the manufacturer is out of stock in their distribution center, it is usually available within a short time. Back orders can last anywhere from a few days to weeks or even months depending upon the reasons for the back order.

Drug products are manufactured from many different sources. If an event occurs that makes the drug resource unavailable, then it may be next to impossible to obtain the raw materials for manufacturing the drug. These days we are hearing of more raw material shortages that are keeping items on back order for longer time periods. A raw material shortage develops when there aren't enough raw materials available for the pharmaceutical companies to produce that particular medication.

If you have a needed item that is on back order, there are certain companies who specialize in hard-to-find items. The price of their products may reflect on this and in turn, the higher purchase prices will increase out of pocket costs for patients.

If the main distribution center for your wholesaler is out-of-stock on an item you need, or perhaps, it is an item that is not stocked in the warehouse facility, it can possibly be drop-shipped to your pharmacy from another location. Sometimes it is necessary and required for items to be drop-shipped from the manufacturer. This is especially true where high cost items as well as those having extraordinary storage requirements are concerned.

For instance, if an item is extremely heavy to ship or cumbersome to store due to size or weight, it may not be feasible for the wholesaler's distribution center to stock the item. Additionally, bulky packaging of items that require refrigeration bring added costs to the wholesaler because not only do they have to have coolers available in which to put such drugs in, they are responsible for paying the costs associated with electricity use to run the refrigerators/coolers.

Returns

There are times when items need to be returned to the wholesaler. Occasionally, an error may have been made during the ordering process and perhaps a wrong drug was requested on the purchase order. Perhaps instead of ordering just 2 bottles of an item, an order for 12 bottles was placed. In these situations and generally speaking, most any item can be returned to the wholesaler for full credit within the first 30 days of purchase.

If the item has been on the shelf for longer than 30 days, it may be that only a partial credit will be given. Still, such a credit would be much better than losing the entire dollar value of the purchase which is what will be the case should the drug expire. 30, 60, 90 and 120 day increments usually decrease the percent of credit that would be offered from the wholesaler to the returning pharmacy. 30-60 days may result in only 95% credit, 60-90 days may drop down to 90%, 90-120 days may not allow but 85% credit and after 120 days on hand, a pharmacy will not likely receive any higher than 80% credit.

The length of time it takes for medication to be ordered, used and then reordered is considered the turnover rate.

The wholesaler will not normally accept expired merchandise for return. Instead, once a drug has expired, it must be returned to the manufacturer for credit. "Big box" return companies can make this process much easier in that they will come in person to the pharmacy, package up those items suitable for return and then handle all the returning process in order for the pharmacy to receive credit from the actual individual manufacturers.

Regardless of return policies, pharmacy stock and inventory turnover rate must be constantly monitored for items that are not moving so that inventory dollars are not sitting on the shelf just waiting to expire. Ideally, the pharmacy's inventory should be turned at least 12 to 14 times a year. If the stock has been sitting on the shelf for more than a few months and no patients are taking that particular medication at that time, it might be worth considering returning it to the wholesaler and reordering it at a later time as it is needed.

National Drug Code

Another aspect of purchasing and inventory control is to consider the NDC number for what it is. This is an identification number that is tagged to that item and that item only. NDC, as well as other pertinent information for new items should be added to the inventory as soon as they are received. The NDC or National Drug Code Number has a standard 5-4-2 format.

The first 5 digits represent the manufacturer. Every product that is made by that manufacturer will have the same first 5 digits. The second 4 digits stand for the drug product. No matter what size package, unit dose or bottle that drug is available in, it will contain the same 4 digits. The last 2 digits signify the size. A bottle of 1000 pills and 100 pills of the same type medication inside would have 2 different digits on the end of the NDC number.

The 5-4-2 format for the NDC makes it standard 11-digit number but oftentimes manufacturers will leave some of the digits off of the printed NDC on the package labeling. If a section of numbers is lacking digits, fill those missing digits in the FRONT of each section with zeros. For example, 12345-6789-01 is a fictitious NDC number entered here only for demonstration purposes. Notice there are 11 digits. However, an additional fictitious NDC number may look something like this: 123-4-56. In this case there are several digits missing. If we add the zeros to fill in the missing spaces, it would look something like this. **00**123-**04**-**00**56. When entering an NDC into the computer for a new drug or other purpose, the 11-digit format should always be used even if it requires adding the missing zeros.

Drug Storage

Proper storage requirements are important. This ensures that the medication is kept under conditions that will keep it fit for use by the patient. At right are some conditions of the environment that affect the safety and efficacy of medications. One consideration of proper storage is the temperature required for the medication. Below is a list of the main temperature storage requirements and their storage temperatures in both Fahrenheit and Celsius degrees.

Some things that affect the safety and efficacy of drugs within the environment are:
* Temperature
* Light
* Humidity
* Packaging

* Room Temperature	59 °F - 86 °F or	15 °C - 30 °C
* Refrigeration	36 °F - 46 °F or	2 °C - 8 °C
* Freezer	< 32 °F or	< 0°C

Always be considerate of storage for pharmaceuticals and mindful of the locations where drugs are stored. For instance, since temperature and humidity greatly affects both safety and efficacy of meds, one should be concerned about where sensitive items are stored. Items like gel caps may not be able to withstand the added heat that the bright fluorescent lights are giving off. Likewise, a bottle of coated tablets may not be able to tolerate being stored near the air conditioning vent due to the humidity that is dispensed there.

Joint Commission Accreditation of Healthcare Organizations is the main organization that does accreditation for health care facilities nationwide. JCAHO requires that different types of medications be stored separately. Orals shouldn't be stored with nasals and otics shouldn't be stored next to the topicals and so on. The group prefers that each "route" has a segregated storage area.

Handling of Hazardous Medications

There are special considerations for working with hazardous materials and some medications fall into this category. JCAHO, OSHA (Occupational Safety and Health Administration) and the NFPA (National Fire Protection Agency) have standards that must be followed when handling hazardous medications and other items. This not only protects the medication from the environment but also protects the healthcare workers and patients from improper use and storage of the medications.

According to the federal hazard communication standard, a hazardous chemical has a physical or health hazard that has been statistically proven to cause acute or chronic health effects in exposed employees. The types of chemicals or substances that may be found in this category include but are not limited to carcinogens, toxins and corrosives. Some items, including certain medications may be considered flammable and therefore may require storage within the walls of an NFPA approved flammable cabinet.

Since the needs of pharmacies will vary, each facility will have its own materials to meet those specific needs. Therefore a unique list of hazardous drugs and other materials for each facility should be created based on specific criteria. If and when a new drug or substance is brought into the pharmacy area, it should be evaluated to see whether it meets the criteria for hazardous materials. If so, it should be handled accordingly and added to the current list of hazardous materials.

All guidelines for the facility should be outlined clearly in the pharmacy's Policy and Procedure manual. Instructions should be in place for all locations and situations in which such drugs and other hazardous materials are handled, used and/or transported throughout the facility. Since such policies would affect more staff than just pharmacy workers, other departments such as nursing, housekeeping, safety, maintenance and other staff may be involved in implementing and enforcing such policies.

Material Safety Data Sheets should be on hand and available for all hazardous materials in the pharmacy area. (unless it is deemed necessary for a specific drug, it is not required to have an MSDS for all medications in the pharmacy) Included in an MSDS sheet would be the handling precautions, Personal Protective Equipment required, damage control and spill management, flammability and other information.

Though the list below is not an all inclusive, it will provide a general idea of the requirements and standards of common policies for handling of hazardous materials.

* MSDS sheets should be available for all hazmat items in the pharmacy.
* Cartons and containers should be visually inspected for possible damage prior to opening during the receiving process.
* Double Gloves should be worn during stocking and handling of hazardous drugs for inventory management. In some cases, gowning may be necessary to handle large or damaged items.
* Hazardous drugs should be stored in segregated areas with shelving barriers that make accidents less likely to happen.
* If refrigeration of hazmat items is required, segregation is required and the items should be contained as in a drawer or compartment to prevent unnecessary contamination should damage occur.
* Distinctive labels should be used on all bins and sealed packaging used to store and transport hazardous drugs to identify potential dangers.
* Spill kits should be readily accessible near hazmat storage areas.
* Eating or drinking should be avoided near hazmat storage areas.
* Hazardous drugs should be clearly labeled at all times during use and transport throughout the facility.

Drug Recalls

Drug recalls are another important aspect of the inventory control. From time to time, the FDA or the manufacturer has a particular reason that medication should be pulled from shelves. Sometimes the recall is voluntarily initiated by the manufacturer because of issues that have presented themselves. Other times, a recall may be initiated and mandated by the FDA due to a potential problem with the drug or its use.

Many recalls are not ever classed and those that are classed are based on the severity of the issue or potential problem. A Class I drug recall involves a health hazard that could possibly result in a serious adverse health consequence or even death. It is the most critical of all drug recalls. A Class II recall has potential for a health hazard with a remote possibility to cause an adverse health consequence. A Class III recall involves a situation in which its use is not likely to cause an adverse health consequence or irreversible damage.

A similar situation with two very different drugs can cause a difference in recall class. Let's say that a drug used for female hormone replacement therapy was being manufactured. Somehow in the process a damp hopper where active and filler ingredient powders were being mixed caused partial contents of active ingredient to remain in the hopper unnoticed. Now the tablets are finished and are in bottles on pharmacy shelves waiting to be dispensed. This is possible even though they lack the total amount of active ingredient that their label states is contained.

166

Is this situation likely to cause irreversible damage to the patient? Probably not, though it may be very uncomfortable for the patient taking those affected tablets. She may be suffering from mood swings, hot flashes and array of other symptoms that coincide with lowered estrogen levels.

Given that same situation but now involving a drug that is used for congestive heart failure, the potential dangers are severely increased. A patient who ends up receiving those affected tablets may not have a chance to report the problem before death is imminent and other patients are affected as well.

The technician can play a major part in purchasing and managing the pharmacy's inventory. This could relieve the burden of this task from the pharmacist's shoulders, giving them more time to spend doing other things. Technicians who are properly trained can do very well placing orders, returning merchandise for credit, adding and removing items from inventory and many other tasks involved in the purchasing and inventory control.

Math Blaster

The calculations used in business management and product pricing are visited in this mission. The mathematics used to calculate the sale prices, percent markups and profit allowance again go back to the simple adding, subtracting, multiplying and dividing. It is simply the matter of knowing how and where to put the numbers.

Calculating Profits and Mark-up

Using the mark-up amount added to the basic acquisition cost allows the determination of profit margins or percentages. If the basic cost of an item is marked up a specific dollar value, the percentage of profit can easily be calculated using the following formula. On the other hand, if a seller wishes to make a certain percent profit on an item, the exact dollar amount can be calculated for the mark-up. Review the examples below.

An item acquired for $8.00 currently sells for $14.29. What percentage is the profit made on this item?

First, determine the mark-up amount. $14.29 - $8.00 = $6.29

Retail price - Cost = Mark-up

Next, divide the mark-up by the cost. $6.29 ÷ $8.00 = 0.79

Mark-up ÷ Cost = Profit

Change the profit from decimal form to a percent. 0.79 ⟶ 79%

A store owner wishes to make a 40% profit on an item that he acquisitioned at $7.29. What is the dollar amount of the mark-up and what would the selling price have to be to ensure such a profit?

First, determine the mark-up amount. $7.29 x 40% = $2.92

Cost   % profit = Mark-up

Next, add mark-up amount to cost. $7.29 + $2.92 = $10.21

Cost   Mark-up   Selling price

168

On another angle, if only the selling price in this situation was needed, the percent profit could simply be added to the cost with a simple click like this:

Add the cost plus the profit percentage. $7.29 + 40% $\longrightarrow$ $10.21

Note when performing calculations with the % key, be careful NOT to use the = sign. The calculation will be done when the % key is pressed.

Discounted Retail Price

If an item is on sale, it may be marked down a specific dollar value. For instance, SAVE $3.00 on these items. However, more commonly done is a discounted percentage. For instance, SAVE 20% off Today ONLY!!! The markdown or discount is taken from the retail or selling price. This markdown is irrelevant to the actual acquisition cost and in most cases that information will not be needed or given in these such calculations. Follow the examples below.

Needing to clear some space, a store owner wishes to offer a 30% savings on specific shelf items in the store. One item was retailed at $8.49. What is the dollar amount of the 30% savings and what would the selling price have to be to ensure such a discount?

First, determine the savings amount. $8.49 x 30%   = $2.55

                                        Cost   % saving   = Discount

Next, subtract discount from selling price. $8.49   - $2.55   = $5.94

                                        Cost   Discount   Selling price

Again if only the selling price in this situation was needed, the discount could simply be subtracted from the cost with a simple click like this:

Subtract the discount from the selling price. $8.49 - 30% $\longrightarrow$ $5.94

Making Change

One of the most common tasks that pharmacy managers feel important for pharmacy technicians to be proficient at is making change when ringing sales up at the cash register. The cash register will actually perform the calculation and show the appropriate amount of change to return to the customer. However, it's up to the technician or cashier (sometimes one and the same) to pull the right amount from the cash drawer and place in the customer's hands. The best way to ensure the correct change is to count the money back from the actual charge of the sale all the way up to the dollar value given.

For instance, if the total sales charge was $13.63 and the customer paid with a $20 dollar bill. That means that $6.37 dollars change should be returned. See the example below on the best way to handle this type of transaction.

$20.00 - $13.63 = $6.37   The register will make this calculation and show amount to be returned to customer. Pull the cash from the drawer and count back in this manner.

$13.63	Charge amount		$14	give 1 quarter
0.64 , 0.65	give 2 pennies		$15	give a 1$ dollar bill
0.75	give 1 dime		$20	give a 5$ dollar bill

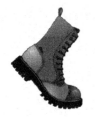

Drill Practice

Complete the following and then check yourself in the rear of the textbook.

Determine the profit margin (percentage) on the following sales.

1. An item that costs $3.00 sells for $4.08. What percent profit is made on each sale of the item?

2. The retail price of a knee brace is $8.56. The acquisition cost of the brace is only $6.86. What percent profit is being made on the sale of the brace?

3. A weight loss supplement currently sells for $18.49 per bottle. The pharmacy pays only $12.00 cost on the product. What is the profit margin earned when someone purchases this item?

4. Strips for a glucometer sell for $42.50 per package. The actual cost of the strips is $36.00. What percent profit is made on this product?

5. An item that currently retails for $99.99 cost the pharmacy only $80.00. What is the profit margin on each sale of this item?

6. The boss wishes to earn a 30% profit on an item that costs $16.86. What would the dollar value of the markup need to be to ensure this amount of profit? What would the actual retail price of the item be?

7. A new bottle of vitamins costs just $12.17. The pharmacy needs to gain 20% profit on the item. What is the markup value? What should the retail price be marked?

8. The pharmacy plans to make 40% profit margin on an item that costs just $2.99. What is the necessary retail price amount for such a profit?

9. A beauty product currently earns the pharmacy a hefty 38% profit margin. If the item costs $21.99 how much does it retail for?

10. A low priced item earns a profit of 60% for the pharmacy. If the acquisition cost sits at $3.29, what is the dollar amount of the markup and what is the actual retail price of the item?

11. A thermometer costs $5.00 and gains a 40% profit. What is it's retail price?

12. A generic store brand pain reliever earns 25% for the pharmacy. It's cost is $3.99 so what would the selling price need to be set at?

13. A bag of adult diapers costs the pharmacy $16.50 and earns a profit of 38%. What is the retail price of the diapers?

14. An item earns a whopping 65% profit but only costs a mere $12.00. What would the selling price need to be to ensure this profit percentage?

15. A shower chair has an acquisition cost of $85.00 but earns a 20% profit for the pharmacy. What is the current retail price of this item?

16. An item currently retailing for $29.99 is on sale at 30% off. What is the new sale price of the item?

17. A discontinued digital blood pressure cuff is being marked down 40%. If it used to retail for $68.99 what is its new price?

18. A daily pill box is on sale this week only for 15% off its regular retail price of $13.76. What would the customer have to pay for this item?

19. A shower chair is on clearance and has a markdown of 90%. The regular retail price was $65.00. How much would the sale price be?

20. An item retailing for $49.99 is being marked down 25%. What is the new discounted price of the item?

21. The total charge of a sale is $12.17. The customer pays with a twenty dollar bill. What is the value of the returned change and how many of which denominations should it be?

$_____

pennies _____ nickels _____ dimes _____ quarters _____

Ones (1$) _____ Fives (5$) _____ Tens (10$)_____ Twenties (20$) _____

22. A patient's bill for meds rings up at $22.15 but all the patient has is a hundred dollar bill. What is the change and how many of which denominations should be given?

$_____ pennies _____ nickels _____ dimes _____ quarters _____

Ones (1$) _____ Fives (5$) _____ Tens (10$)_____ Twenties (20$) _____

23. A sale for $3.62 is paid for with a five dollar bill. How much change and in what denominations should be given in return?

$_____ pennies _____ nickels _____ dimes _____ quarters _____

Ones (1$) _____ Fives (5$) _____ Tens (10$)_____ Twenties (20$) _____

24. A customer owes $60.19 for all purchases and hands the cashier four twenties. What is the value of the change and of which denominations should the customer receive?

$_____ pennies _____ nickels _____ dimes _____ quarters _____

Ones (1$) _____ Fives (5$) _____ Tens (10$)_____ Twenties (20$) _____

25. A batch of prescriptions totals $49.82 and a patient pays with a hundred dollar bill. What amount should be returned and in which denominations?

$_____ pennies _____ nickels _____ dimes _____ quarters _____

Ones (1$) _____ Fives (5$) _____ Tens (10$)_____ Twenties (20$) _____

Drug Training Chapter Seven

Brand Name	Generic Name	Drug Classification	Primary Indication	Side effects, Warnings, Other
Klonopin	Clonazepam	Benzodiazepine	Panic Disorder, Seizure prevention	Drowsiness, ataxia, somnolence, depression, asthenia, depression
Chantix	Varenicline	Smoking Deterrent	Smoking Cessation Therapy	May increase risk of depression, suicidal ideation and attempted/completed suicide; May also cause nausea, abnormal dreams, constipation, flatulence, and vomiting
Lasix	Furosemide	Diuretic	Edema of various causes	GI disturbances, tinnitus, parasthesia, dizziness, orthostatic hypotension
Celexa	Citalopram	Selective Serotonin Reuptake Inhibitor	Depression	May increase risk of suicidal thinking and behavior, nausea, dry mouth, ejaculation disorder, fatigue
Lamictal	Lamotrigine	AntiConvulsant	Seizure treatment/ prevention, Bipolar disorder	May cause serious rash; dizziness, ataxia, somnolence, headache, diplopia, blurred vision, nausea, vomiting, rash
Lipitor	Atorvastatin	Lipid-lowering	Reduce cholesterol levels	Nasopharyngitis, arthralgia, diarrhea, pain in extremity, and UTI
Dilaudid	Hydromorphone	C II Opioid Analgesic	moderate to severe pain where opioid anagesia is appropriate	light-headedness, dizziness, sedation, nausea, vomiting, sweating, dysphoria, euphoria, dry mouth, and pruritus.
Skelaxin	Metaxalone	Skeletal Muscle Relaxant	Acute, painful musculoskeletal conditions	Drowsiness, dizziness, headache, nervousness, nausea, vomiting, gastrointestinal upset.

Brand Name	Generic Name	Drug Classification	Primary Indication	Side effects, Warnings, Other
Lotensin	Benazepril	ACE inhibitor	Hypertension	Headache, dizziness, fatigue, cough
Estrace	Estradiol	Sex Hormone	Estrogen Replacement therapy in post-menopausal women; osteoporosis prevention for high risk patients	May increase risk of myocardial infarction, stroke, breast and endometrial cancers and blood clots; also may cause various changes in menses, breast tenderness/enlargment, GI upset
Benicar	Olmesartan	Angiotensin II Receptor Blocker (ARB)	Hypertension	Chest pain, peripheral edema, vertigo, dyspepsia, arthralgia, myalgia, rash
Zocor	Simvastatin	Lipid-lowering Agent	Reduce cholesterol levels	May cause myopathy manifested as muscle pain, tenderness or weakness with creatine kinase (CK) above ten times the upper limit of normal (ULN).

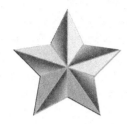

Mission 7 Debriefing

Answer the following questions in assessment of the lessons learned in Mission 6. For best results, repeat the exercise until no questions are missed then move on to the next mission.

1. Which two documents can be used to track purchases?
    a) Packing slip and invoice
    b) Purchase order and packing slip
    c) MSDS and invoice
    d) Purchase order and invoice

2. Generally speaking, scheduled 2 (C II) controlled substances are stored _____.
    a) Under additional lock and key such as in a safe, vault, cabinet or drawer.
    b) On the pharmacy shelves with other routine pharmaceuticals
    c) In a "special" area on the pharmacy shelf devoted to controlled substances
    d) None of these

3. When receiving and checking the order in, this should be done in an area away from the main flow of traffic primarily to deter theft especially of controlled substances.
    a) True
    b) False

4. Which of the following pairs of medications are lipid lowering agents?
    a) Lotensin and Benicar
    b) Chantix and Klonopin
    c) Lipitor and Zocor
    d) Celexa and Chantix

5. An item that costs $2.00 sells for $4.54. What percent profit is made on each sale of the item?
    a) 1.27%
    b) 12.7%
    c) 2.5%
    d) 127%

6. An NDC number has a specific numerical format of 5-4-2.
    a) True
    b) False

7. Which of the pharmaceuticals below can be ordered without having any special paperwork other than submitting a purchase order to the vendor?
    a) OTC items
    b) Non-controlled legend drugs
    c) C III - V controlled substances
    d) Any and all of these

8. What is the proper storage temperature for an item to be kept in the freezer?
    a) Less than 32° C
    b) Less than 32° F
    c) Less than 36° F
    d) Less than 5° C

9. How may we submit the DEA form 222C to the wholesaler for request of C II pharmaceuticals?
   a) Hand deliver it
   b) Fax it
   c) Email it
   d) Mail it
   e) Any of these
   f) Only b and c
   g) Only a and d
   h) Only c and d

10. To confirm receipt of all invoiced items, a line by line invoice check should be performed.
    a) True
    b) False

11. Dilaudid is a _____ opioid analgesic medication.
    a) C II
    b) C III
    c) C IV
    d) C V

12. Strips for a glucometer sell for $58.75 per package. The actual cost of the strips is $40.00. What percent profit is made on this product?
    a) 19%
    b) 47%
    c) 21%
    d) 32%

13. The process of stock rotation involves placing received items on the shelf with _____.
    a) earliest expirations are at the back.
    b) earliest expirations are at the front.
    c) latest expiration dates are at the front
    d) none of these

14. Ordering direct from each individual manufacturer is more popular than using group purchasing organizations or large wholesalers for supplying pharmaceuticals in today's world.
    a) True
    b) False

15. Which copy of the DEA222C form remains on file with the wholesaler after the order has been filled and shipped to the requesting pharmacy?
    a) Original copy 1 (white)
    b) Copy 2 (green)
    c) Copy 3 (blue)
    d) No copies remain on file there

16. Which of the following medications is used in smoking cessation therapy?
    a) Celexa
    b) Chantix
    c) Skelaxin
    d) Lotensin

17. In the NDC number of 12345-6789-01, what does the 12345 represent?
    a) Manufacturer
    b) Drug product
    c) Package size
    d) Lot number

18. CSOS, the newer way to request C II pharmaceuticals, is also known as _____.
    a) Controlled Substances Online Supply
    b) Controlled Substances Online Submission
    c) Controlled Substances Ordering Supply
    d) Controlled Substances Ordering System

19. An item to be stored at room temperature should be kept at _____.
    a) 36 °F - 46 °F
    b) 59 °F - 86 °F
    c) 2 °C - 8 °C
    d) None of the above

20. Proper inventory management requires effort from the entire pharmacy team.
    a) True
    b) False

21. The manager wishes to earn a 40% profit on an item that costs $12.76. What would the dollar value of the markup need to be to ensure this amount of profit?
    a) $17.86
    b) $5.10
    c) $22.96
    d) $25.00

22. The want book is simply a list of things that need to be placed on the order at the end of the day.
    a) True
    b) False

23. Lasix is classified as a(n)_____.
    a) skeletal muscle relaxant
    b) SSRI
    c) ACE inhibitor
    d) diuretic

24. Which of the following classes of controlled substances have more potential for abuse and therefore are more difficult to procure or acquisition?
    a) C IIs
    b) C IIIs
    c) C IVs
    d) C Vs

25. Generally speaking, most any item can be returned to the wholesaler within 30 days of purchase for full credit.
    a) True
    b) False

26. When receiving the order, which of these need to be reported to the wholesaler as soon as possible?
    a) Expired items
    b) Damaged items
    c) Shorted items
    d) All of these

27. A patient's bill for meds rings up at $24.85 but all the patient has is a hundred dollar bill. What denominations should be given as change?
    a) 3 twenty dollar bills, 1 five dollar bill, 1 dime and 1 nickel
    b) 3 twenty dollar bills, 1 ten dollar bill, 1 five dollar bill, 1 dime and 1 nickel
    c) 2 twenty dollar bills, 1 ten dollar bill, 1 five dollar bill, 1 dime and 1 nickel
    d) 3 twenty dollar bills, 1 ten dollar bill, 1 dime and 1 nickel

28. If flammable items are kept in the pharmacy, regulations may require that they are stored in an NFPA approved flammable cabinet.
    a) True
    b) False

29. Which of the following pairs of medications are indicated for hypertension?
    a) Simvastatin and atorvastatin
    b) Olmesartan and benazepril
    c) Citalopram and clonazepam
    d) Lamotrigine and varenicline

30. Storing items on pharmacy shelves could be done in _____ order.
    a) alpha-brand
    b) alpha-generic
    c) alphabetical
    d) any of these are common

31. In the NDC number of 12345-6789-01, what does the 6789 represent?
    a) Manufacturer
    b) Drug product
    c) Package size
    d) Lot number

32. Expired drugs can be returned to the wholesaler for partial credit.
    a) True
    b) False

33. Ideally, a pharmacy's inventory turnover should occur at least _____ times per year.
    a) 7 – 10
    b) 10 – 12
    c) 12 – 14
    d) 14 – 20

34. The triplicate DEA222C form used to order C II controlled substances must not have any errors or overmarkings to remain valid.
    a) True
    b) False

35. A beauty aid night cream currently earns the pharmacy a hefty 36% profit margin. If the item costs $24.00 how much does it retail for?
    a) $42.64
    b) $8.64
    c) $15.36
    d) $32.64

36. Which of the following is a benefit of using the CSOS for acquiring C II scheduled drugs?
    a) Unlimited items on a single PO
    b) Next day delivery
    c) No preprinted forms needed
    d) All of these

37. Estradiol may be prescribed when patients are at a high risk for _____.
    a) myocardial infarction
    b) myopathy
    c) osteoporosis
    d) suicidal thinking

38. MSDS sheets should be available for all hazardous materials in the pharmacy area.
    a) True
    b) False

39. An item needs to be stored under refrigeration. It should be kept at _____.
    a) 2 °C - 8 °C
    b) 15 °C - 30 °C
    c) 36 °F - 46 °F
    d) Both a and b
    e) Both a and c
    f) None of these

40. When controlled substances are concerned the purchase order is proof of receipt.
    a) True
    b) False

41. An ear thermometer is on sale this week only for 10% off its regular retail price of $89.99. What would the customer have to pay for this item?
    a) $8.99
    b) $80.99
    c) $7.29
    d) $7.99

42. If an error is made and a DEA222C form is voided it can be shredded and discarded.
    a) True
    b) False

43. Since all medications can be dangerous if used improperly, an MSDS sheet must be available for each and every drug in stock.
    a) True
    b) False

44. A customer owes $60.49 for all purchases and hands the cashier three twenties and a ten dollar bill. What change should the customer receive?
    a) 3 five dollar bills, 1 quarter, 2 dimes and 4 pennies.
    b) 1 ten dollar bill, 2 quarters, 1 penny
    c) 1 five dollar bill, 4 one dollar bills, 2 quarters and 1 penny
    d) 1 ten dollar bill, 1 quarter 2 dimes and 4 pennies

45. Which of the following medications is an ACE inhibitor?
    a) Lotensin
    b) Lasix
    c) Lamictal
    d) Lipitor

46. What information would be found on an MSDS sheet?
    a) Handling precautions
    b) PPE requirements
    c) Damage control
    d) Spill management
    e) Flammability
    f) All of these

47. If the manufacturer distribution center is out of stock on an item and is unable to ship that item out to the wholesaler(s), this is referred to as _____.
    a) temporarily out of stock
    b) manufacturer's back order
    c) drop shipment required
    d) none of these

48. In the event of an audit by a third party payor such as Medicaid, Medicare or other private insurance payor, yielding of any invoices, purchase orders and other related documents is necessary and required.
    a) True
    b) False

49. Clonazepam is a _____ controlled substance.
    a) C II
    b) C III
    c) C IV
    d) C V

50. A contract with a primary wholesaler or prime vendor in which a pharmacy promises to purchase the majority of their pharmaceuticals is often referred to as a _____.
    a) wholesaler contract
    b) prime vendor agreement
    c) sales agreement
    d) price break

51. A low priced item earns a profit of 70% for the pharmacy. If the acquisition cost sits at $2.80 what is the dollar amount of the markup?
   a) $4.76
   b) $0.84
   c) $3.64
   d) $1.96

52. Which of the following pairs of medications place patients at a higher risk of suicidal thinking/behavior?
   a) Chantix and Dilaudid
   b) Celexa and Chantix
   c) Celexa and Lamictal
   d) Chantix and Skelaxin

53. A potty chair has an acquisition cost of $82.00 but earns a 25% profit for the pharmacy. What is the current retail price of this item?
   a) $102.50
   b) $92.50
   c) $61.50
   d) $20.50

54. Which of the following reasons might cause an item to be returned to the wholesaler?
   a) The item is no longer being used.
   b) The wrong drug was ordered by mistake.
   c) Too many bottles were ordered in error.
   d) Any of these could require a return.

55. After receiving the DEA222C from the pharmacy, it is filled and the original white copy is forwarded on to the DEA office by the wholesaler.
   a) True
   b) False

56. A patient has been diagnosed with depression. Which of these meds below has likely been prescribed?
   a) metaxalone
   b) lamotrigine
   c) simvastatin
   d) citalopram

57. The most severe of all classed recalls is a _____.
   a) Class I
   b) Class II
   c) Class III
   d) Both a and c

58. When storing invoices for pharmaceuticals, which of the following should be filed separately?
   a) OTC and legend items
   b) C III – C V items
   c) C II items
   d) All of these

59. The pharmacy technician can play a major role in purchasing and inventory management.
   a) True
   b) False

60. In the NDC number of 12345-6789-01, what does the 01 represent?
   a) Manufacturer
   b) Drug product
   c) Package size
   d) Lot number

61. Mrs. Smithson has been having muscle spasms and her doctor has prescribed a skeletal muscle relaxant. Which of the following may have been the drug prescribed?
    a) Varenicline
    b) Atorvastatin
    c) Metaxalone
    d) Benazepril

62. Temperature, light, humidity and packaging can greatly affect the efficacy of a medication.
    a) True
    b) False

63. A drug call must be initiated by the manufacturer of the drug being recalled.
    a) True
    b) False

64. Guidelines for pharmacy ordering procedures will generally be found in the _____.
    a) MSDS book
    b) Policy and Procedures Manual
    c) Want book
    d) None of these

65. Where handling hazardous materials is concerned, which of the following statements is true?
    a) It is not necessary to store these items segregated from other stock.
    b) A single pair of latex gloves will prevent exposure to hazmat substances.
    c) Hazardous materials should never be stored in the refrigerator.
    d) Eating or drinking should not be done in the area hazmat items are stored.

66. A lift chair has been put on clearance with a markdown of 70%. The regular retail price was $586.99 so what is the newly advertised sale price?
    a) $293.50
    b) $410.89
    c) $997.88
    d) $176.10

67. When a pharmaceutical product passes its expiration date, it must be returned to _____ for any possible credit to be issued.
    a) the FDA
    b) the manufacturer
    c) the primary wholesaler
    d) no credit given for expired products

68. With a purchasing contract in place with a primary vendor, a pharmacy generally promises to purchase _____ of their pharmaceuticals in order to gain better purchase pricing.
    a) 60-70%
    b) 70-80%
    c) 80-90%
    d) 90-100%

69. What are some likely reasons for items being drop-shipped from the manufacturer rather than being shipped with the wholesale order?
    a) Items have a high acquisition cost.
    b) Items have extraordinary storage requirements
    c) Items are extremely heavy or have bulky packaging making shipping costs higher.
    d) All of these are likely reasons for drop-shipment.

70. Who is eligible to apply for and receive a digital certificate and electronic signature code from the DEA office for "signing" the CSOS orders for controlled substances?
    a) Technicians
    b) Pharmacists
    c) Both a and b
    d) Neither a nor b

182

71. The FDA requires that different routes of drugs (i.e. orals, injectables, topicals) be stored separately.
    a) True
    b) False

72. If given the following NDC number, 425-23-1, which of the following would be correct in the proper 11-digit format?
    a) 42500-23-10
    b) 42500-23-01
    c) 00425-23-10
    d) 00425-0023-01

73. Which agencies have standards that must be followed when handling hazardous pharmaceuticals and other hazardous substances?
    a) OSHA
    b) NFPA
    c) JCAHO
    d) All of these

74. Which of the following recall classes is the least likely to cause an adverse health consequence.
    a) Class I
    b) Class II
    c) Class III
    d) None of the above

75. When a wholesaler is out of an item but expecting a shipment soon from the manufacturer, this could be referred to as _____.
    a) drop shipment
    b) manufacturer back order
    c) backstock
    d) temporarily out of stock

76. Which of the following pairs of medications may be used in helping prevent seizures?
    a) Lipitor and Zocor
    b) Klonopin and Lamictal
    c) Benicar and Lotensin
    d) Dilaudid and Celexa

Match the following drugs to their generic names.

77. Zocor   _____ a) simvastatin
78. Estrace   _____ b) olmesartan
79. Klonopin   _____ c) lamotrigine
80. Lasix   _____ d) atorvastatin
81. Skelaxin   _____ e) clonazepam
82. Lipitor   _____ f) varenicline
83. Lamictal   _____ g) estradiol
84. Dilaudid   _____ h) benazepril
85. Benicar   _____ i) citalopram
86. Lotensin   _____ j) furosemide
87. Celexa   _____ k) hydromorphone
88. Chantix   _____ l) metaxalone

Match the following drugs to their classifications.

89. Clonazepam   _____ a) Angiotension Receptor Blocker
90. Citalopram   _____ b) C II opioid analgesic
91. Hydromorphone   _____ c) anticonvulsant
92. Estradiol   _____ d) lipid lowering agent
93. Simvastatin   _____ e) diuretic
94. Benazepril   _____ f) hormone replacement
95. Atorvastatin   _____ g) lipid lowering agent
96. Furosemide   _____ h) SSRI
97. Varenicline   _____ i) smoking deterrent
98. Lamotrigine   _____ j) skeletal muscle relaxant
99. Metaxalone   _____ k) ACE inhibitor
100. Olmesartan   _____ l) C IV benzodiazepine

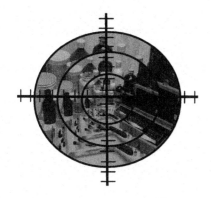

Mission 8
The Nervous System
Medications and Malfunctions

Mission Objectives

*To understand the basic anatomy and physiology of the nervous system.

*To identify the functions of organs that comprise the central nervous system.

*To comprehend the autonomic nervous system and its functions.

*To learn of the drug families used in treating nervous system disorders.

 *To understand the pharmacology of drugs used in treating nervous system disorders.

*To gain baseline knowledge of twelve of the most popular drugs on the market.

*To review oral dosage calculations, day supply, dispense quantities and DEA number validation.

The **nervous system** is, by far, the most important and complex of all body systems. The body cannot function properly on its own without a healthy nervous system. Nearly all other body systems would be useless if the nervous system did not do its job. It receives and relays information from outside the body and inside the body to cause the correct signals to be sent to appropriate glands, muscles and other body parts so coordinated responses can be produced.

The nervous system has two main divisions. First, the **central nervous system**, otherwise known as **CNS**, consists of the **brain, spinal cord** and **motor** and **sensory nerves** which lead to and from the spinal cord. The other part is the **autonomic nervous system**, or **ANS**. The ANS, in turn, is also broken down into two divisions. These are called **sympathetic** and **parasympathetic**. Both CNS and ANS are vital to normal body function, but they are very different and serve different purposes.

Central Nervous System

The CNS controls all voluntary function. The main organ of the CNS is the brain. It weighs about three pounds and is gray in color. The largest section of the brain is the **cerebrum**. The **cerebral cortex**, or outer layer, contains billions and billions of nerve cells. These nerve cells, also called **neurons**, control conscious mental activity.

Deep inside the cerebrum, far below the gray wrinkles of the cerebral cortex, lay two very important structures. The **thalamus** coordinates information received from the eyes, ears, mouth, and skin and relays that information to the higher places in the brain. Take note that these are the sensory organs and help to produce the sensations we feel when we sense things. Directly below and much smaller than the thalamus lies the **hypothalamus**. This tiny structure controls hunger, thirst, shivering, perspiration and many other essential processes.

The **cerebellum** lies below and behind the larger cerebrum. It is responsible for monitoring information from muscles, tendons, joints and inner ear; then, it acts to bring about muscular movements upon instruction of the cerebrum to do so. The **medulla oblongata** is found at the top of the spinal cord where it gets slightly larger. Here in the medulla are vital reflex centers involved in controlling such functions as heart rate, blood pressure and respiration.

The neurons have one or more fibers varying in length. Some are less than an inch, others might be 3 feet or longer; depending on their location and function. The longer nerve fibers are called **axons** and carry nerve impulses away from the cell body. The shorter fibers, known as **dendrites**, bring impulses to the cell body. These neurons follow the nerve pathway like a domino effect. One neuron signals the next and so on. As the nerve impulse reaches a junction or synapse, it releases a chemical substance at the nerve ending. This chemical substance acts like a bridge between two neurons; therefore, the impulse can be carried on down the nerve pathway.

Sensory neurons carry impulses directly through the spinal cord to the brain. These impulses produce the sensations we feel like heat, cold, sight, sound, touch, pain and pressure. The sensory neurons relay this information to the brain through sensory receptors. Each of these receptors responds only to its own kind of signals.

The **motor neurons** carry signals from the brain and/or spinal cord to the tissues and muscles all over the body. The fibers of these motor neurons end in motor end plates that are very close to the muscle fibers. When the impulse gets to the motor end plate, the nerve ending releases acetylcholine. This chemical substance acts like a neurotransmitter to bring about muscle cell activity. As the muscle contracts an enzyme called **cholinesterase** starts to clear away the **acetylcholine** to make ready for the next impulse.

The neurons are more active than other body cells; therefore they use more oxygen and glucose than other cells do. We are born with all the neurons we will ever have. The small number that die out each day are so few that the body doesn't notice, but those that die out cannot be replaced.

Autonomic Nervous System

The autonomic nervous system controls the automatic functions of the body. The control of smooth muscle tissue, of internal organs and glandular secretions are in this division of ANS. The two branches of this complex part of the nervous system are sympathetic (**adrenergic**) and parasympathetic (**cholinergic**). Both of these branches of the ANS are two-neuron systems. The first being the preganglionic neuron begins within the CNS and ends outside the CNS at the ganglion, which is a cluster of nerve cell bodies. The second neuron starts at the ganglion and ends at the tissue it is meant to act upon.

The two systems work together by doing the exact opposite of each other. The **sympathetic system** is in control when the body is under stress. This system usually has an excitatory effect on the body. This sympathetic branch of ANS is sometimes referred to as the "fight or flight" system. It releases chemical signals called neurotransmitters to stimulate organs that are needed when we are excited or stressed, such as the heart and lungs. It also suppresses bodily functions that are not vital during a time of stress.

Acetylcholine and norepinephrine work as neurotransmitters for the sympathetic system. Acetylcholine acts to bridge the synapse from the preganglionic neuron to the postganglionic neuron. Norepinephrine works between the postganglionic neuron and the tissue receptor.

The adrenergic receptors are:

* $Alpha_1$
* $Alpha_2$
* $Beta_1$
* $Beta_2$.

The **$Alpha_1$** receptors are located in smooth muscle tissue of peripheral blood vessels, in the urinary bladder, in male sex organs and many other tissues. When they are stimulated, the result is constricted blood vessels, a constricted sphincter in the bladder and normal ejaculatory function in males along with other physiological reactions. **$Alpha_2$** receptors are presumed to be on the presynaptic neuron to control the release of neurotransmitters. If these receptors are stimulated, the neurotransmitter's release is reduced. **$Beta_1$** receptors are primarily located in the muscles of the heart and fatty tissue. Their stimulation brings about increased heart rate. **$Beta_2$** receptors are mainly found in bronchial smooth muscle. Stimulating $Beta_2$ receptors causes bronchodilation.

Sympathetic nerves run parallel to the spinal cord on either side. They are linked to the spinal cord along the length of it but not at either end. The parasympathetic system arises from both ends of the spinal cord. It also releases neurotransmitters that affect mostly the same organs that are affected by the sympathetic system; only the effect is much different.

The parasympathetic system has a reverse response on the body. The neurotransmitters that are released by this division have a calming effect on the body to slow it down. When the body is at rest the **parasympathetic system** steps up to the plate and takes control. This branch promotes energy conservation by reducing heart rate and blood pressure. It helps nutrient utilization by increasing gastricmovement and secretion of gastric acids. It also helps to enhance waste elimination due to increased muscular tone in the intestines and bladder.

Acetylcholine is one of the neurotransmitters of the parasympathetic system. There are two types of acetylcholine receptors. Those in postganglionic portion are referred to as muscarinic receptors. The receptors, which are located at the ganglia sites as well as the neuromuscular junction of the motor neurons, are called nicotinic receptors since they respond to nicotine.

In summary, the nervous system is, by far, the most important and complex of all body systems. It's because the nervous system controls the other body systems in one way or another.

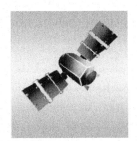

Recon Mission 8:

There are so many different diseases that can be associated with the nervous system. With this mission's reconnaissance you are encouraged to search the Internet for information on various diseases and disorders of the nervous system and also seek out anatomical diagrams of the nervous system so that each area becomes more familiar to you now that a review of the functionality has been completed. Many websites offer interactive diagrams which allow you to label and maneuver them.

Write down as many of the conditions as you can find with a brief description of each one. As you continue on this mission, some medications may be discussed that are used primarily to treat diseases and disorders that you have read about and familiarized yourself with. As a guide only, the following bulleted points could be used as keywords in your search. Each keyword suggested below may have multiple possible inclusions for your review. You are encouraged to devote plenty of time to this activity.

* Nervous System diseases and disorders
* Psychosis
* Mental illnesses
* Interactive diagrams of the Nervous System, Brain and Nerves

---

Medications for Malfunctions

There are many drug classes that affect the nervous system. Remember that the nervous system has two major divisions of CNS and ANS. Here in this mission the medications affecting the Central Nervous System will be reviewed while those medications which affect the various areas falling within the Autonomic Nervous System will be reviewed in the individual missions to follow. Here you will learn of the basic classes and their pharmacological actions on the body. Take into consideration that true pharmacology goes much deeper than you will learn in this preparatory course, but you should obtain enough information to understand the basic actions on the body for these medications.

Cholinesterase Inhibitors are indicated for patients with Alzheimer's disease or who are suffering from dementia problems. These medications increase the concentration of acetylcholine through reversible inhibition of its breakdown by acetylcholinesterase.

* Aricept – Donepezil
* Exelon – Rivastigmine
* Razadyne ER - Galantamine

Skeletal muscle relaxants are used in the treatment of musculoskeletal conditions. These may be a result of pulled or strained muscles or a chronic disease like Multiple Sclerosis, which affects muscle function. Baclofen is more likely to be used in chronic conditions whereas cyclobenzaprine is a commonly used muscle relaxant for treatment of acute muscle spasms. All that are listed below are centrally acting agents.

* Flexeril – Cyclobenzaprine
* Lioresal – Baclofen
* Robaxin – Methocarbamol
* Soma – Carisoprodol
* Zanaflex - Tizanidine

Most **barbiturates** are mainly used for the sedative-hypnotic effects. Phenobarbital and mephobarbital are more often used for their anti-convulsant effects. Barbiturates produce all levels of CNS depression depending on the dosing. This class of medications depresses the sensory cortex, decreases motor activity, alters cerebullar function and produces drowsiness, sedation and hypnosis. For these reasons, this class of medications is often used during sedation for various surgeries and/or other procedures where a level of relaxation needs to take place.

There are other sedative-hypnotics that do not belong to the barbiturate family. Zolpidem is a well known non-barbiturate sedative. Its actions are similar to those of benzodiazepines. Several of the benzodiazepines are primarily used for their sedative-hypnotic effects. You will find them included in the list below.

* Mebaral – Mephobarbital   **Barbiturates**
* Nembutal - Pentobarbital
* Seconal – Secobarbital
* Dalmane – Flurazepam   **Benzodiazepines**
* Restoril – Temazepam
* Noctec - Chloral Hydrate   **Other sedative - hypnotics**
* Rozerem – Ramelteon
* Sonata – Zaleplon
* Ambien – Zolpidem
* Lunesta - Eszopiclone

Though a few "benzo"s as they are familiarly known, are mainly used for sleep induction, many anti-anxiety agents are **benzodiazepines.** These drugs potentiate the effects of GABA (gamma-amino butyrate) by binding to specific benzodiazepine receptor sites. Lower doses produce anxiolytic effects while ataxia and sedation occur at doses beyond those needed for anxiety treatment. Therefore there are various uses for this drug family.

Hydroxyzine is an **anti-anxiety agent** that is not a benzodiazepine. It is a rapid-acting calmative. It induces a calming effect in anxious, tense, and psychoneurotic adults without impairing mental alertness. Most all anti-anxiety agents have potential for causing drowsiness, but usually after several days of treatment the body develops a tolerance to the medication and this drowsiness dissipates.

* Ativan - Lorazepam   **Benzodiazepines**
* Xanax – Alprazolam
* Klonopin – Clonazepam
* Tranxene – Chlorazepate
* Valium - Diazepam
* Vistaril – Hydroxyzine Pamoate   **Other**
* Atarax – Hydroxyzine HCl
* Buspar – Buspirone
* Sinequan – Doxepin

NSAID's (Non Steroidal Anti-Inflammatory Drugs) are used to treat pain and inflammation usually associated with the joints, although you will see them used for many different types of mild to moderate pain. Some are available for purchase without a prescription. NSAID's are believed to inhibit cyclooxgenase(COX). There are two COX isoenzymes that have been identified, referred to as COX-1 and COX-2.

The majority of NSAIDs inhibit both COX-1 and COX-2. Therefore, the stomach is more likely to produce ulcers, due to the inhibition of prostaglandin synthesis. The latest NSAIDs, such as celecoxib are known as **COX-2 inhibitors** and offer a much lesser chance of stomach irritation and ulcer formation. All NSAIDs including the COX-2 inhibitors should be taken with food. The first dose of the drug ketorolac is generally given via IM injection and then followed by oral treatment not to exceed 5 days worth of medication. Dosing is normally four times daily.

* Indocin – Indomethacin
* Motrin – Ibuprofen
* Naprosyn – Naproxen
* Toradol – Ketorolac
* Celebrex – Celecoxib   **COX -2 inhibitor**

Anti-Depressants known as **tricyclics** have a triple pharmacologic action, thus the classification as a tricyclic. They block the amine pump, cause sedation and also cause peripheral/central anticholinergic action. They also inhibit the reuptake of seratonin and norepinephrine. Some anti-depressants are known as SSRIs or Selective Seratonin Reuptake Inhibitors. These particular drugs inhibit the reuptake of seratonin with a weak effect on norepinephrine and dopamine reuptake and little effect on anything else. Other antidepressants are referred to as SNRIs or Seratonin and Norepinephrine Inhibitors. The most common side effect of all anti-depressants is sedation and anticholinergic effects.

*	Elavil – Amitriptyline	**Tricyclics**
*	Pamelor – Nortriptyline	
*	Tofranil – Imipramine	
*	Celexa – Citalopram	**SSRIs**
*	Paxil - Paroxitine	
*	Prozac – Fluoxetine	
*	Zoloft – Sertraline	
*	Cymbalta – Duloxetine	**SNRIs**
*	Effexor – Venlafaxine	
*	Pristiq- Desvenlafaxine	
*	Desyrel – Trazadone	**Others**
*	Serzone – Nefazadone	
*	Wellbutrin – Buproprion	

Parkinsonism is believed to be caused from an imbalance of neurotransmitters: too much acetylcholine and not enough dopamine. **Anti-Parkinson agents**, which are centrally acting anticholinergic agents like work to diminish the tremors associated with Parkinson's. Other agents such as levodopa are known as dopaminergic agents. Since levodopa is a precursor of dopamine and directly increases the content of dopamine in the brain; it is currently the most effective treatment for Parkinsonism. Since many antipsychotic medications cause Parkinson-like side effects, patients who are taking those medications may also be given an AntiParkinson agent to help alleviate some of the effects of the antipsychotic meds.

* Artane – Trihexyphenidyl
* Congentin – Benzatropine
* Parlodel – Bromocriptine
* Sinemet – Carbidopa/Levodopa

Anti-psychotic symptoms are usually grouped into two categories. These are positive ones which include delusions, disorganized speech, hallucinations and behavior disturbances and negative ones such as social withdrawal. Mechanism of action in most **anti-psychotic agents** is unclear. Pharmacotherapy is aimed at improving the target symptoms while maintaining the most tolerable side effect at the lowest possible dose. Side effects of anti-psychotic medications include Parkinson-like symptoms of tremors and drooling, involuntary movements of the face, muscle spasms in neck, and a constant condition of motor restlessness.

*	Thorazine – Chlorpromazine	**Phenothiazines**
*	Compazine – Prochlorperazine	
*	Stelazine – Trifluoperazine	
*	Mellaril - Thioridazine	
*	Clozaril – Clozapine	**Dibenzapines**
*	Loxitane - Loxapine	
*	Zyprexa – Olanzapine	
*	Seroquel - Quetiapine	
*	Navane – Thiothixene	**Other**
*	Haldol - Haloperidol	
*	Risperdal – Risperidone	
*	Geodon – Ziprasidone	
*	Abilify – Aripiprazole	
*	Eskalith – Lithium Carbonate	

Anti-Convulsants are used in the treatment and prevention of seizures. The mechanism of action in most anti-convulsants is not known. Maintaining a certain blood level of the anti-convulsant medication is best prevention for seizures. It is important to try to keep patients on the same brand of medications that they have received in the past. Switching brands often may affect the blood levels and therefore increase chance for having seizures. Some benzodiazepines, though used in other disease states, are also used for their anticonvulsant properties.

* Depakote – Valproic Acid
* Dilantin – Phenytoin
* Gabitril - Tiagabine
* Keppra Levetiracetam
* Lamictal – Lamotrigine
* Neurontin – Gabapentin
* Tegretol – Carbemazepine
* Trileptal - Oxcarbazepine
* Topamax – Topiramate

Acetaminophen, like many other medications, wears two hats. It is both an **antipyretic** and an **analgesic.** This means it relieves pain with its analgesic properties but also reduces fever with its antipyretic properties by direct action on the hypothalamic heat-regulating center, which increases dissipation of body heat through sweating and vasodilatation.

Narcotic analgesics and Narcotic analgesic combinations work by their activity on opioid receptors. Their use has a known side effect of nausea. This nausea is caused by directed stimulation of the emetic chemoreceptors in the medulla. This class of medications should be taken with food and it's quite common that they would cause drowsiness and constipation.

* Demerol – Meperidine
* Duragesic Patch – Fentanyl
* Lortab, (Lorcet, Vicodin) - Hydrocodone /Acetaminophen
* Tylenol – Acetaminophen
* Tylenol #3 – Acetaminophen/Codeine
* Ultram – Tramadol
* Vicoprofen - Hydrocodone w/Ibuprofen

Anti-emetics are indicated for nausea, vomiting, motion sickness, and vertigo (dizziness). When the emetic chemoreceptors have been stimulated, they stimulate the vomiting center. This stimulation occurs when there is increased activity of the neurotransmitters. (Dopamine in the chemoreceptor trigger zone/Acetylcholine in the vomiting center). Anti-dopaminergics such as promethazine and prochlorperazine are more effective for drug-induced nausea. On the other hand, anticholinergics like dimenhydrinate and meclizine work better for normal motion sickness and vertigo.

The newest class of antiemetics, 5-HT_3 receptor antagonists, are favorable with many patients as they traditionally cause fewer side effects than the older generation drugs.

* Compazine – Prochlorperazine	**AntiDopaminergics**
* Phenergan – Promethazine	
* Thorazine - Chlorpromazine	
* Antivert – Meclizine	**AntiCholinergics**
* Dramamine – Dimenhydrinate	
* Anzemet – Dolasetron	**5-HT_3**
* Kytril – Granisetron	**Receptor Antagonists**
* Zofran – Ondansetron	

CNS stimulants such as methylphenidate and amphetamine salts are indicated for treatment of ADD and ADHD. There are other indications but this are the most common ones. Patients on this class of medications are monitored closely and must return back often to see their prescribers. The majority of these medications are C II controlled substances and cannot be written with refills. In addition, weight loss is monitored due to the possibility of appetite suppression which is the main side effect with use of these type drugs. The lateral hypothalamic feeding center is believed to be the site for appetite suppression.

* Ritalin – Methylphenidate
* Dexadrine – Dextroamphetamine

Disulfiram is an anti-alcoholic medication. It is used in the management of sobriety in chronic alcoholics. Effectiveness is limited to compliance. The interaction with alcohol reaction produces flushing, throbbing, nausea and copious vomiting, respiratory difficulty and confusion among other things. A "No Alcohol" auxiliary label should be affixed to a prescription for this medication.

* Antabuse - Disulfiram

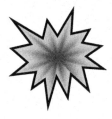

Math Blaster

For the Mission 8 Math Blaster, feel free to review the explanations in Mission 3 for the pharmacy calculations. In the mission 8 debriefing, you will be revisiting the skills learned in the earlier Mission.

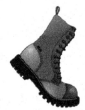

Drill Practice

For this mission's drill practice, rework those questions found in Mission 3 drill practice. In the mission 8 debriefing, you will be checking to see how well you remember those skills.

Drug Training Chapter Eight

Brand Name	Generic Name	Drug Classification	Primary Indication	Side effects, Warnings, Other
Flonase	Fluticasone	Intranasal Steroid	Rhinitis, sinusitis	Headache, GI upset, epistaxis, pharyngitis, rhinorrhea
Cipro	Ciprofloxacin	Fluoroquinolone Anti-Bacterial Agent	Treatment of susceptible infections in adults 18 years of age and older.	May increase risk of tendinitis and tendon rupture in all ages; ciprofloxacin therapy were nausea, diarrhea, abnormal liver function tests, vomiting and rash
Bactrim	Sulfamethoxazole /Trimethoprim	Sulfa-derivative Anti-Bacterial Agent	treat susceptible strains of infection including those otitis media, UTI,URI	nausea, vomiting, allergic skin reactions such as rash and urticaria
Nasonex	Mometasone	Intranasal Steroid	Seasonal and perennial allergic rhinitis	Headache, viral infection, upper respiratory disturbances
Duragesic	Fentanyl (transdermal patch)	C II Opioid Analgesic	Persistant moderate to severe chronic pain unrelieved by other opioid treatments	Used in opioid tolerant patients may cause respiratory depression, fever, nausea & vomiting and/or drowsiness
Flexeril	Cyclobenzaprine	Skeletal Muscle Relanxant	Acute, painful musculoskeletal conditions	Drowsiness, dizziness, mouth, fatigue, GI disturbances
Protonix	Pantoprazole	Proton Pump Inhibitor	Esophagitis, Gastroesophageal Reflux Disease (GERD)	Headache, GI upset, facial edema
Januvia	Sitagliptin	Dipeptidyl peptidase-4 (DPP-4) inhibitor	Type 2 Diabetes	Hypoglycemia, nasopharyngitis, upper respiratory infection and disturbances, headache

Brand Name	Generic Name	Drug Classification	Primary Indication	Side effects, Warnings, Other
Imdur	Isosorbide Mononitrate	Nitrate Vasodilator	Angina	Headache, Dizziness, Nausea
Zyprexa	Onlanzapine	Anti-Psychotic Agent	Schizophrenia, Bipolar I Disorder,	Note: Elderly patients with dementia-related psychosis treated with antipsychotic drugs are at an increased risk of death; may cause somnolence, weight gain, and peripheral edema, dizziness, dry mouth, asthenia
Cartia XT	Diltiazem	Calcium Channel Blocker	Hypertension	edema, headache, dizziness, asthenia, bradycardia, flushing, nausea and rash
Lioresal	Baclofen	Muscle Relaxant, Anti-spastic	Spasticity or muscle rigidness due to Multiple Sclerosis	Note: Not indicated for acute skeletal muscle spasm from rheumatic disorders; May cause transient drowsiness, dizziness, weakness, fatigue

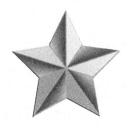

Mission 8 Debriefing

Answer the following questions in assessment of the lessons learned in Mission 8. For best results, repeat the exercise until no questions are missed then move on to the next mission.

1. The central nervous system and the autonomic nervous system are very similar in action and functionality.
   a) True
   b) False

2. When _____ receptors are triggered or stimulated bronchodilation occurs.
   a) Alpha$_1$
   b) Alpha$_2$
   c) Beta$_1$
   d) Beta$_2$

3. _____ are indicated for patients suffering from Alzheimer's or other dementia related illnesses.
   a) NSAIDs
   b) COX-2 inhibitors
   c) Barbiturates
   d) Cholinesterase inhibitors

4. The first dose of ketorolac is generally given via IM injection and then followed by oral treatment up to QID not to exceed _____ worth of medication.
   a) 30 days
   b) 10 days
   c) 7 days
   d) 5 days

5. Switching brands often of anticonvulsant medications puts patients at higher risk for seizure activity and therefore should be avoided whenever possible.
   a) True
   b) False

6. All of the following are SSRI antidepressants except _____.
   a) Cymbalta
   b) Paxil
   c) Zoloft
   d) Celexa

7. Narcotic analgesic combinations include an opioid analgesic combined with either acetaminophen or ibuprofen. Which of the following are narcotic analgesic combination medications?
   a) Lortab
   b) Tylenol #3
   c) Vicoprofen
   d) All of these

8. The _____ relays information from the sensory organs to the brain.
   a) cerebellum
   b) cerebrum
   c) thalamus
   d) hypothalamus

9. Which of the following anxiety agents is a benzodiazepine agent?
   a) Diazepam
   b) Doxepin
   c) Duloxetine
   d) None of these

10. How many vials of insulin will a patient taking 45 units sq q am and 12 units q pm need for at least 30 days supply?
    a) 4 vials
    b) 3 vials
    c) 2 vials
    d) 1 vial

11. The majority of CNS stimulants indicated for ADD and ADHD are _____ and cannot be written with refills available.
    a) C II
    b) C III
    c) C IV
    d) C V

12. Phenytoin is an antipsychotic medication.
    a) True
    b) False

13. _____ neurons produce sensations such as heat, cold, sight, sound, touch, pain and pressure.
    a) Dendrite
    b) Axon
    c) Motor
    d) Sensory

14. Ibuprofen is a COX-2 inhibitor.
    a) True
    b) False

15. A patient has dropped off a prescription for a pain medication that cannot be refilled under any circumstances. Which of these medications must it have been written for?
    a) Protonix
    b) Duragesic
    c) Cartia XT
    d) Flexeril

16. Most all anti-anxiety agents have potential for causing _____, but usually after several days of treatment the body develops a tolerance and this condition dissipates.
    a) drowsiness
    b) nausea
    c) headaches
    d) heartburn

17. There are several different classification groups of antidepressants including trycyclics, SSRIs and SNRIs.
    a) True
    b) False

18. One of the chemical substances that creates a bridge between two neurons is _____.
    a) cholinesterase
    b) adrenergase
    c) nicotine
    d) acetylcholine

198

19. Flexeril is commonly used to treat acute cases of muscle spasm.
    a) True
    b) False

20. Though many barbiturates are used as sedative-hypnotics, Phenobarbital and Mephobarbital are primarily used as _____ agents.
    a) Anti-anxiety
    b) Anti-depressant
    c) Anti-convulsant
    d) Anti-psychotic

21. A prescription is dropped off at the pharmacy window. It reads: Lactulose syrup 2 Tbsp bid for 30 days. What amount of lactulose syrup should be dispensed?
    a) 600mL
    b) 1800mL
    c) 900mL
    d) 1200mL

22. The drug _____ is a COX – 2 inhibitor.
    a) Motrin
    b) Celebrex
    c) Toradol
    d) Indocin

23. Which of the following is controlled by the medulla oblongata?
    a) Heart rate
    b) Respirations
    c) Blood pressure
    d) All of these

24. The most effective treatment for parkinsonism are products containining _____.
    a) Levodopa
    b) Benzatropine
    c) Venlafaxine
    d) None of these

25. The cerebellum contains billions of neurons which control conscious mental activity.
    a) True
    b) False

26. Elderly patients with dementia-related psychosis may be at increased risk of death if treated with which of these drugs below?
    a) Zyprexa
    b) Lioresal
    c) Cipro
    d) Januvia

27. When Alpha$_1$ receptors are stimulated the peripheral blood vessels become constricted.
    a) True
    b) False

28. A patient presents a script for Prednisone 5mg tablets with the following directions.
    ii po tid x2 days, then i po tid x2 days, then i po bid x2 days, i po qd x2 days then stop. Calculate the number of tablets needed to fill the order.
    a) 24 tablets
    b) 120 tablets
    c) 18 tablets
    d) 36 tablets

29. NSAIDS are mainly used to treat _____.
    a) Nausea and vomiting
    b) Constipation
    c) Pain and inflammation
    d) Edema and swelling

30. The cerebellum monitors information from the muscles, tendons, joints and inner ear to bring about muscular movements when necessary.
   a) True
   b) False

31. Which of the following pairs of medications are antibacterial agents?
   a) ciprofloxacin and cyclobenzaprine
   b) sitagliptin and sulfamethoxazole/trimethoprim
   c) baclofen and cyclobenzaprine
   d) ciprofloxacin and sulfamethoxazole/trimethoprim

32. The hypothalamus controls _____.
   a) hunger
   b) thirst
   c) perspiration
   d) shivering
   e) Only a and b
   f) All of these

33. Which of the following is a cholinesterase inhibitor?
   a) Carisoprodol
   b) Donepezil
   c) Secorbarbital
   d) Zaleplon

34. An antipyretic agent reduces _____.
   a) Pain
   b) Blood pressure
   c) Fever
   d) Appetite

35. Zolpidem is a well known non-barbiturate sedative.
   a) True
   b) False

36. _____ is an antialcoholic medication used in managing sobriety.
   a) Methylphenidate
   b) Granisetron
   c) Disulfiram
   d) Fentanyl

37. The _____ system promotes energy conservation by reducing heart rate and blood pressure.
   a) sympathetic
   b) parasympathetic

38. COX-2 inhibitor NSAIDS should offer a lesser chance of _____.
   a) Pain in the extremities
   b) Drowsiness
   c) Stomach irritation and ulcers
   d) Dizziness or vertigo

39. Which of these agents indicated for nausea and vomiting are found in the newer classification 5-HT$_3$ Receptor Antagonists?
   a) Phenergan
   b) Kytril
   c) Zofran
   d) Compazine
   e) Both b and c
   f) None of these

40. How many days will a 6oz bottle of cough syrup last that is dispensed with the following directions? Take 1 teaspoonful by mouth every 8 hours.
   a) 4 days
   b) 5 days
   c) 7 days
   d) 12 days

41. Methylphenidate is a(n) _____.
    a) Antidepressant
    b) Antianxiety agent
    c) CNS stimulant
    d) Anti-alcoholic agent

42. Which of the following pairs of medications are SNRI antidepressants?
    a) Effexor and Prestiq
    b) Paxil and Prozac
    c) Celexa and Zoloft
    d) All of these are SNRIs

43. Axons are shorter nerve fibers which bring impulses toward the cell body.
    a) True
    b) False

44. Circle the only possible valid DEA # for Dr. Ritchings from the choices below.
    a) AD2873644
    b) AR 3826786
    c) BR1249009
    d) BD3482798

45. Clozaril is an antipsychotic agent.
    a) True
    b) False

46. The sympathetic system, a division of the ANS, can also be referred to as _____.
    a) parasympathetic
    b) cholinergic
    c) dendraegic
    d) adrenergic

47. Buspirone is classed as an_____.
    a) antianxiety agent
    b) antidepressant
    c) anticonvulsant
    d) antipsychotic

48. Baclofen is used more in treating acute conditions with muscle pain.
    a) True
    b) False

49. The drug pantoprazole is classified or known as a(n) _____.
    a) antibacterial
    b) muscle relaxant
    c) proton pump inhibitor
    d) calcium channel blocker

50. If a patient gets the following prescription from a doctor, how much medication should be dispensed?

    Prelone syrup 5mg/5mL

    Give i tsp po tid x 3 days, then i tsp bid x 3 days, then

    i tsp qd x 3 days, then stop.

    a) 18mL
    b) 60mL
    c) 180mL
    d) 90mL

51. Lioresal and Flexeril are both _____.
    a) opioid analgesics
    b) skeletal muscle relaxants
    c) antibacterials
    d) steroids

52. A patient's insulin regimen consists of 70 units each morning and 45 units each evening. How many days will each vial last the patient?
    a) 12 days
    b) 9 days
    c) 8 days
    d) 7 days

53. All of the following are anti-convulsants except _____.
    a) gabapentin
    b) levetiracetam
    c) oxcarbazepine
    d) quetiapine

54. A patient that is a newly diagnosed schizophrenic may be taking which of these for his condition?
    a) Zyprexa
    b) Cartia XT
    c) Protonix
    d) Januvia

55. How many 60mg doses are in a 120mL bottle of clindamycin 75mg/5mL?
    a) 20 doses
    b) 16 doses
    c) 30 doses
    d) 24 doses

56. Anti-emetics are indicated for _____.
    a) Pain and inflammation
    b) Fever
    c) Appetite suppression
    d) Nausea and vomiting

57. Aripiprazole is an antidepressant agent.
    a) True
    b) False

58. Which of the following patient age groups should not be taking the drug ciprofloxacin?
    a) Under 2 years
    b) Under 12 years
    c) Under 18 years
    d) Over 60 years

59. Which of the following pairs of drugs are intranasal steroids?
    a) pantoprazole and cyclobenzaprine
    b) fentanyl and baclofen
    c) ciprofloxacin and cyclobenzaprine
    d) fluticasone and mometasone

60. A patient gives the pharmacy a prescription for cephalexin 250mg , ii po tid. If 60 capsules will be dispensed, what will be the days supply for this prescription?
    a) 7 days
    b) 10 days
    c) 14 days
    d) 20 days

61. The drug Cipro may increase the risk of _____.
    a) suicidal thoughts
    b) tendonitis
    c) myocardial infarction
    d) death

62. The pharmacist takes a call in script from the local clinic. As you are keying the data in for preparing the dispensing label, you must calculate the amount to dispense. The script reads: Cefdinir 300mg po bid for 7 days. The pharmacy only stocks the 250mg/5mL. How much will be needed?
    a) 70mL
    b) 120mL
    c) 84mL
    d) 98mL

63. If a patient was allergic to sulfa agents, which of these should he/she not be taking?
   a) Cartia XT
   b) Cipro
   c) Januvia
   d) Bactrim

64. The drug Isosorbide Mononitrate is classed or known as a(n) _____.
   a) calcium channel blocker
   b) vasodilator
   c) fluoroquinolone
   d) analgesic

65. A patient has just been prescribed a calcium channel blocker. Which of these may have been written for that patient?
   a) Pantoprazole
   b) Diltiazem
   c) Fentanyl
   d) Cyclobenzaprine

66. Which of the following could not possibly be a valid DEA number for Dr. Frances Swearingen?
   a) BS2436841
   b) FS4399970
   c) AS2253869
   d) BS2688438

67. Which of the following substances work as sympathetic neurotransmitters?
   a) Acetylcholine
   b) Norepinephrine
   c) Both a and b
   d) Neither a nor b

68. Anticonvulsants are used in the treatment and prevention of seizures.
   a) True
   b) False

69. How many 20mEq doses can a patient take from a 12oz of potassium elixir containing 10mEq/15mL?
   a) 12
   b) 24
   c) 4
   d) 8

70. Tricyclic antidepressants have triple action pharmacology. Which of the antidepressants below are from the tricyclic classification?
   a) Pamelor
   b) Elavil
   c) Tofranil
   d) All of these

71. An _____ reduces or relieves pain.
   a) Analgesic
   b) Antipyretic

72. When _____ receptors are triggered or stimulated the heart rate increases.
   a) Alpha$_1$
   b) Alpha$_2$
   c) Beta$_1$
   d) Beta$_2$

73. Anti-psychotic pharmacotherapy is aimed at which of the following _____.
   a) Improving target symptoms
   b) Using the lowest dose possible
   c) Maintaining tolerable side effects
   d) All of these

74. The drug Sinemet is most often used to treat patients who suffer from _____.
   a) muscular dystrophy
   b) Alzheimer's
   c) Parkinson's
   d) nausea

75. Which of these medications are skeletal muscle relaxants?
   a) Carisoprodol and cyclobenzaprine
   b) Ibuprofen and Nalbuprofen
   c) Tizanidine and baclofen
   d) Both a and b
   e) Both a and c
   f) Both b and c

76. Which of the following sedative-hypnotics are benzodiazepines?
   a) Restoril
   b) Ambien
   c) Seconal
   d) Lunesta

Match the following drugs to their generic names.

77. Imdur   _____ a) baclofen
78. Protonix   _____ b) fluticasone
79. Lioresal   _____ c) pantoprazole
80. Flonase   _____ d) sitagliptin
81. Cartia XT   _____ e) diltiazem
82. Bactrim   _____ f) isosorbide mononitrate
83. Flexeril   _____ g) mometasone
84. Zyprexa   _____ h) ciprofloxacin
85. Cipro   _____ i) cyclobenzaprine
86. Duragesic   _____ j) onlanzapine
87. Nasonex   _____ k) sulfamethoxazole/trimethoprim
88. Januvia   _____ l) fentanyl

Match the following drugs to their classifications.

89. Fluticasone   _____ a) Intranasal steroid
90. Sulfamethoxazole/Trimethoprim _____ b) C II opioid analgesic
91. Baclofen   _____ c) fluoroquinolone
92. Mometasone   _____ d) DPP-4 inhibitor
93. Fentanyl   _____ e) antispasmodic muscle relaxant
94. Pantoprazole   _____ f) proton pump inhibitor
95. Sitagliptin   _____ g) intranasal steroid
96. Isosorbide Mononitrate   _____ h) sulfa derivative antibacterial
97. Diltiazem   _____ i) calcium channel blocker
98. Cyclobenzaprine   _____ j) skeletal muscle relaxant
99. Ciprofloxacin   _____ k) antipsychotic agent
100. Onlanzapine   _____ l) vasodilator

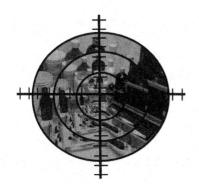

Mission 9
The Gastrointestinal System
Medications and Malfunctions

Mission Objectives

*To understand the basic anatomy and physiology of the gastrointestinal system.

*To learn of the drug families used in treating gastrointestinal disorders.

*To understand the pharmacology of drugs used in treating digestive disorders.

*To gain baseline knowledge of twelve of the most popular drugs on the market.

*To review injectable dosage calculations and dosing by weight.

The gastrointestinal system or digestive system is one of the major systems of the body. This awesome system breaks down the food we eat into chemical components that can be used to continue the process of life. This system is primarily made up of smooth, involuntary muscle tissue in the form of a tube with openings on each end. The entrance, being the mouth, where the food is taken in and the exit, being the anus, where waste products are passed outside the body. In the middle is where the magic of the digestive process takes place.

To begin this process, the body takes in food to eat. It is chewed by the teeth to become swallowable. While food is being chewed, the salivary glands are releasing saliva, which starts the conversion of starches into simple sugars. As swallowing takes place, three things happen simultaneously. As the tongue pushes the food to the back of the mouth, the soft palate rises to block the nasal cavity. At the same time, the epiglottis covers the opening of the trachea or windpipe. The esophagus opening relaxes and accepts the incoming food to be further digested. The esophagus is the section of the digestive system that connects the mouth to the stomach. It is lined by mucous and has thin walls, which consist of both skeletal and smooth muscle tissue. These muscles contract and relax causing movement of the food on into the stomach. This muscle action, called peristalsis, occurs not only in the esophagus, but also throughout the remainder of the gastrointestinal system.

The esophagus joins the stomach and the place where the two organs meet is generally closed. It is kept closed by a ring of muscles called the cardiac sphincter. The only time it relaxes is when food needs to enter the stomach. When the stomach receives food, its muscular walls begin to contract in a way that helps to mix up the food. It also releases gastric enzymes, primarily pepsin, to inhibit further digestion and absorption of the food. Pepsin breaks down protein, but it needs hydrochloric acid (also produced by the stomach) to do its job. This acid is strong enough to burn skin, yet the mucous-coated walls of the stomach protect this organ from its own secretions.

As food and gastric juices are mixed up, they form a mixture known as chyme. From this chyme, substances such as water, glucose, alcohol, salts and other electrolytes can be readily absorbed when it reaches the small intestine. This chyme enters the small intestine through an opening called the pyloric sphincter. This movement happens at a rate of about one percent per minute.

The small intestine is where the majority of digestion and absorption does occur. It is the longest section of the gastrointestinal system. This one organ is broken down into 3 sections, which are the duodenum, the jejunum and the ileum. It is made up of smooth muscle tissue that continues the peristalsis action. This mixes the chyme with additional enzymes to further the breakdown process.

In the duodenum, or first section, is where some of these additional enzymes are received. The pancreatic juices come from the pancreas, of course. Bile is produced by the liver, but it is stored in the gall bladder until it is needed. While food is in this first section, fat, carbohydrates and proteins are all broken down where they can be absorbed by the body. Bile salts use the churning movement of the duodenum to break large fat droplets into smaller ones. Then lipase and bile salts can break down fats to even tinier droplets called micelles.

Meanwhile, amylase, another enzyme is beginning the breakdown of carbohydrates to dextrose and maltose. Two more enzymes, trypsin and chymotrypsin are released while the food mixture is still in the duodenum. These two break down proteins into simple amino acids.

The middle section of the small intestine, known as the jejunum, is where much of the absorption takes place. Tiny finger-like projections called villi lie inside the jejunum walls. These villi are what absorb most of the food mixture. Villi are able to absorb through a network of capillaries and microvilli located on or under the surface. Intestinal glands situated at the base of the villi release enzymes that help to complete the digestion process. The mixture of food aided by digestive juices is now broken down into simple substances that can be used by the body.

The food now moves by peristalsis into the last section of the small intestine known as the ileum. This section is filled with a thick lining of villa that will finish this stage of absorption before pushing the remaining chyme into the colon.

The colon, or large intestine, is the last major portion of the gastrointestinal system. It is shorter than the small intestine, but much larger in diameter. It joins the ileum in the lower right abdomen. This area of the colon is called the cecum.

Attached to the cecum, dangling vertically is the appendix. This small organ has little known value to the body. The appendix may become infected with bacteria, which causes it to become inflamed. This will ultimately result in surgical removal of the appendix. This has no effect on the digestive process.

When food reaches the colon, digestion and absorption are almost finished. What's left to be absorbed or passed on is, primarily undigestable roughage, dead cells, salts and water. Major changes happen to the remains of the food substance at this point.

Friendly bacteria feed on the waste products and change it to feces. The bacteria also produce valuable vitamins and more enzymes, which are absorbed along with water and some salts through the wall of the colon.

This process happens as the waste travels up the ascending colon, through the transverse colon and descending colon before entering the section called the sigmoid colon. After this, the rectum holds the feces until the body pushes it through an opening called the anus.

Thus, this concludes the digestive process. The body is now using its other complex systems to use what has just been absorbed to benefit the body as a whole.

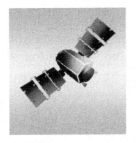

Recon Mission 9:

There are so many different diseases that can be associated with the gastrointestinal system. With this mission's reconnaissance you are encouraged to search the Internet for information on various diseases and disorders of the GI system and also seek out anatomical diagrams of the GI system so that each area becomes more familiar to you now that a review of the functionality has been completed. Many websites offer interactive diagrams which allow you to label and maneuver them.

Write down as many of the conditions as you can find with a brief description of each one. As you continue on this mission, some medications may be discussed that are used primarily to treat diseases and disorders that you have read about and familiarized yourself with. As a guide only, the following bulleted points could be used as keywords in your search. Each keyword suggested below may have multiple possible inclusions for your review. You are encouraged to devote plenty of time to this activity.

* Gastrointestinal System diseases and disorders
* Digestive illnesses
* Interactive diagrams of the Gastrointestinal System

Medications for Malfunctions

There are many drug classes that affect the Gastrointestinal system. Here you will learn of the basic classes and their pharmacological actions on the body. Take into consideration that true pharmacology goes much deeper than you will learn in this preparatory course, but you should obtain enough information to understand the basic actions on the body for these medications.

H$_2$ Antagonists block histamine at the H$_2$ receptors. They are effective in alleviating symptoms and help to prevent complications of Peptic Ulcer disease. Once available by prescription only, all of this drug family is now available for purchase over the counter. The target indication has evolved into relief from day to day heartburn and indigestion from gastric acid.

* Tagamet - Cimetidine
* Zantac - Ranitidine
* Pepcid - Famotidine
* Axid   - Nizatidine

Proton Pump inhibitors suppress gastric acid secretion by specific inhibition of systemic enzyme referred to as the acid (Proton) pump. Proton Pump inhibitors block the final step of acid production and in doing so they provide relief for patients who are suffering from Gastroesophageal Reflux Disease. Several of these PPI drugs are now FDA approved for over the counter sales. Prilosec OTC was the leader of the over the counter PPIs being the first available to provide self-treatment.

* Prilosec – Omeprazole
* Prevacid – Lansoprazole
* Nexium – Esomeprazole
* Aciphex – Rabeprazole
* Protonix - Pantoprazole

Antacids neutralize gastric acidity, resulting in increased PH of the stomach. Though antacids do not suppress gastric secretions, they are indicated for similar conditions as other meds which do. Indications ranging from indigestion, heartburn, acid reflux are common with these drugs though their effectiveness is limited to short-term relief. Most antacids can be bought without a prescription.

* Maalox , Mylanta - Magnesium hydroxide/ Aluminum Hydroxide
* Tums – Calcium Carbonate

Anticholinergic/Antispasmodic medications act to decrease motility in the GI tract which slows down the digestion process. These drugs inhibit muscarinic actions of acetylcholine at postganglionic neuroeffector sites.

* Levbid– Hyoscyamine
* Bentyl – Dicyclomine
* Robinul - Glycopyrrolate

Laxatives function by promoting active electrolyte secretion, decreasing water and electrolyte absorption, or increasing hydrostatic pressure in the gut. Laxatives cause stimulation in the bowel which can trigger the urge for bowel movement. Other meds that are very mild to the GI system are stool softeners. Though the plain stool softeners do not necessarily have stimulant properties, they do help to keep the bowels moving regularly.

* Dulcolax – Bisacodyl
* Chronulac – Lactulose
* Colace – Docusate Sodium
* Senokot – sennosides

Anti-diarrheals promote bulk density in the bowel. They slow down intestinal motility and help to diminish the loss of fluids. Some are prescription only, while others can be bought over the counter.

* Lomotil – Diphenoxylate/Atropine
* Imodium - Loperamide

Anti-flatulents have a foaming action that relieves flatulence (gas) by dispersing and preventing the formation of "mucous surrounded" gas pockets. Most drugs in this family are available without a prescription.

* Mylicon - Simethicone

GI stimulants increase the motility of the GI tract without stimulating GI secretions. These medications help to empty the bowel quicker in patients with conditions resulting in delayed gastric emptying.

* Reglan - Metoclopramide

A good point to remember is that laxatives decrease water absorption and stimulate motility in the bowel, while

anti-diarrheals increase water absorption and decrease motility in the gut.

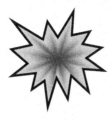 **Math Blaster**

For the Mission 9 Math Blaster, feel free to review the explanations in Mission 4 for the pharmacy calculations. In the mission 9 debriefing, you will be revisiting the skills learned in the earlier Mission.

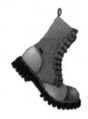 **Drill Practice**

For this mission's drill practice, rework those questions found in Mission 4 drill practice. In the mission 9 debriefing, you will be checking to see how well you remember those skills.

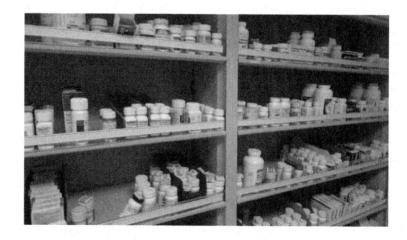

Drug Training Chapter Nine

Brand Name	Generic Name	Drug Classification	Primary Indication	Side effects, Warnings, Other
Calan SR	Verapamil	Calcium Channel Blocker	Hypertension, Angina or Arrythmias	Constipation, nausea, headache, dizziness, edema, hypotension
Levoxyl, Synthroid	Levothyroxine	Thyroid	Hypothyroidism	Symptoms of hypothyroidism can occur including fatigue, increased appetite or weight loss, heat intolerance, fever, excessive sweating, headache, dysnea, hyperactivity, anxiety, irritability, insomnia, tremors, arrhythmias, GI upset
Bactroban	Mupirocin	Topical anti-infective	Impetigo and other skin infections	burning, stinging, pain,itching
Valium	Diazepam	C IV Benzodiazepine	management of anxiety disorders or for short-term relief of anxiety	drowsiness, fatigue, muscle weakness, and ataxia
Relafen	Nabumetone	Non-Steroidal Anti-inflammatory Drug (NSAID)	Osteoarthritis and Rheumatoid Arthritis	May increase risk of cardiovascular thrombotic events, myocardial infarction, stroke and GI bleeding; may also cause diarrhea, dyspepsia, and abdominal pain.
Minocin	Minocycline	Tetracycline Derivative Antibacterial	Treatment of susceptible strains of infection	Avoid dairy products or antacids, may cause secretion discoloration, GI upset, photosensitivity
Thyroid, (Armour)	Thyroid	Thyroid hormone replacement	Hypothyroidism, Thyroid Stimulating Hormone Suppression	Adverse reactions other than those indicative of hyperthyroidism due to therapeutic overdosage are rare

Brand Name	Generic Name	Drug Classification	Primary Indication	Side effects, Warnings, Other
Biaxin	Clarithromycin	Macrolide AntiBacterial Agent	Susceptible strains of various infections	Diarrhea, nausea, abnormal taste, dyspepsia, abdominal pain/discomfort, and headache
Aldactone	Spironolactone	Potassium Sparing Diuretic	Hypertension, Edema, Hyperaldosteronism	Drowsiness, lethargy, Abdominal cramping
Glucotrol	Glipizide	Sulfonylurea	Type 2 Diabetes	Gastrointestinal disturbances, skin reactions, anemia
Compazine	Prochlorperazine	AntiEmetic, AntiPsychotic, Tranquilizer	Nausea and Vomiting, Schizophrenia, generalized non-psychotic anxiety	Drowsiness, dizziness, amenorrhea, blurred vision, skin reactions and hypotension
Vibramycin, Doryx Vibratab	Doxycycline	Tetracycline-derivative anti-bacterial agent	Various strains of susceptible infection	Avoid dairy products or antacids; may cause photosensitivity and reduce effectiveness of contraceptives; May also cause GI upset, rash

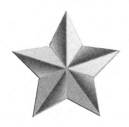

Mission 9 Debriefing

Answer the following questions in assessment of the lessons learned in Mission 9. For best results, repeat the exercise until no questions are missed then move on to the next mission.

1. As food is swallowed, what happens simultaneously?
   a) The soft palate rises.
   b) The esophagus opening relaxes.
   c) The epiglottis covers the trachea.
   d) All these things happen at once.

2. What holds the feces until a bowel movement occurs?
   a) Anus
   b) Colon
   c) Rectum
   d) Sigmoid

3. Prochlorperazine is available in a 5mg/mL 5mL MDV. A physician has ordered 12.5mg q6h prn nausea post chemotherapy treatments for a patient on the oncology ward. What volume of medication should be administered to achieve the ordered dose?
   a) 0.4mL
   b) 1.25mL
   c) 2.5mL
   d) 4mL

4. Glipizide is indicated for _____.
   a) infection.
   b) diabetes
   c) hypertension
   d) hyperthyroidism

5. With the assistance of hydrochloric acid, _____ begins the breakdown of proteins into simply amino acids where they can be absorbed and used for energy.
   a) Bile
   b) Lipase
   c) Amylase
   d) Pepsin

6. H_2 antagonists can be purchased without a prescription.
   a) True
   b) False

7. The digestive system is primarily comprised of _____ muscle tissues.
   a) striated
   b) smooth
   c) involuntary
   d) voluntary
   e) Both a and d
   f) Both b and c

8. The large intestine is the longest section of the gastrointestinal system.
   a) True
   b) False

9. In the _____ most of the absorption of nutrients occurs during digestion.
   a) Ileum
   b) Duodenum
   c) Jejunum
   d) Colon

10. Digestion starts in the _____.
    a) mouth
    b) esophagus
    c) stomach
    d) small intestine

11. Which of the following pairs of medications are used to treat patients who suffer from hypothyroidism?
    a) Calan SR and Aldactone
    b) Biaxin and Vibramycin
    c) Relafen and Compazine
    d) Levoxyl and Armour Thyroid

12. If 750mg dose of medication needs to be given q8h, what volume will need to be drawn from the stock vial if it contains 150mg/mL?
    a) 0.2mL
    b) 1.6mL
    c) 2.5mL
    d) 5mL

13. The villi are able to absorb most of the nutrients from the gut through a network of capillaries and microvilli on or under the surface.
    a) True
    b) False

14. The drug Nabumetone make cause increased risk of _____.
    a) constipation
    b) cardiovascular events
    c) photosensitivity
    d) suicidal thinking

15. Trazodone has a recommended dosing of 1.5-2mg/kg/day given in equally divided doses qid. A patient weighing 176lbs has been placed on this medication. What will the range of each dose need to be to remain within recommended manufacturer's guidelines?
    a) 80-120mg
    b) 90-110mg
    c) 30-40mg
    d) 80-120mg

16. GI stimulants decrease the motility of the gastrointestinal tract.
    a) True
    b) False

17. Which of the following medications are indicated for bacterial infection?
    a) Vibramycin
    b) Minocin
    c) Biaxin
    d) All of these

18. A cancer patient is suffering from nausea after a recent treatment and her physician has approved a one time injection of chlorpromazine. The ordered dose is 30mg IM STAT. If the medication is stocked in a 25mg/mL SDV what volume should be administered to the patient?
    a) 6mL
    b) 4.2mL
    c) 1.2mL
    d) 0.8mL

19. Proton pump inhibitors suppress gastric acid secretion.
    a) True
    b) False

20. The _____ connects the mouth to the stomach.
    a) pancreas
    b) esophagus
    c) gall bladder
    d) trachea

21. Though verapamil and spironolactone are from different drug families, they both are indicated for _____.
    a) hypertension
    b) hypothyroidism
    c) anxiety
    d) pain

22. What volume of a 80mg/2 mL gentamycin injection will deliver a dose of 64 mg which needs to be administered?
    a) 1.25mL
    b) 0.6mL
    c) 1.6mL
    d) 2.5mL

23. Aciphex is an H_2 antagonist available for over the counter purchase.
    a) True
    b) False

24. In the duodenum, bile salts and lipase break down _____.
    a) proteins into amino acids
    b) carbohydrates into simple sugars
    c) fats into micelles
    d) electrolytes into simple salts

25. A patient has just been prescribed Lactulose for a current condition. The patient needed a(n) _____.
    a) antacid
    b) antidiarrheal
    c) antiflatulant
    d) laxative

26. The physician has recently ordered an antibiotic injectable for a patient who weighs in at 132lbs. The appropriate dosage is 50mg/kg q8h. How many milligrams would be given each time?
    a) 1000mg
    b) 60mg
    c) 300mg
    d) 3g

27. A patient has been suffering with nausea and vomiting and her physician has ordered an antiemetic for some relief. Which of the following drugs may have been prescribed?
    a) Prochlorperazine
    b) Doxycycline
    c) Minocycline
    d) Spironolactone

28. Which of the drugs below could have been prescribed for a patient needing drug with an antispasmodic effect on the bowel?
    a) Dicyclomine
    b) Docusate
    c) Nizatidine
    d) Simethicone

29. The brand name for the drug glycopyrrolate is _____.
    a) Lomotil
    b) Raglan
    c) Robinul
    d) Bentyl

30. Aldactone is a non-potassium sparing diuretic.
    a) True
    b) False

31. Which of the following are H₂ antagonists?
    a) Aciphex
    b) Axid
    c) Tums
    d) Nexium

32. Prilosec OTC was the first proton pump inhibitor available without a prescription.
    a) True
    b) False

33. A sedative recommended for children is to be given at 2-6mg/kg/day in 3 or 4 equal doses. Generally recommendations of this nature result in starting with lower doses and titrating up if necessary. The patient has a weight of 66 lbs. What will the range of dosing be if giving QID?
    a) 20-60mg
    b) 15-45mg
    c) 60-180mg
    d) 30-40mg

34. In the duodenum, trypsin and chymotrypsin break down _____.
    a) proteins into amino acids
    b) carbohydrates into simple sugars
    c) fats into micelles
    d) electrolytes into simple salts

35. The ileum is the last section of the small intestine.
    a) True
    b) False

36. Which of the following may increase risk of photosensitivity?
    a) Vibramycin
    b) Minocin
    c) Vibratab
    d) All of these

37. Biaxin is a _____ antibacterial agent.
    a) tetracycline derivative
    b) penicillin derivative
    c) fluoroquinolone
    d) macrolide

38. Laxatives do which of the following pharmacologic actions?
    a) Promote electrolyte secretion
    b) Increase hydrostatic pressure in the gut
    c) Decrease water absorption
    d) All of these

216

39. Bactroban is a(n) _____ preparation.
    a) otic
    b) topical
    c) injectable
    d) inhaled

40. Peristalsis is the action that occurs which moves the food mixture throughout the gut.
    a) True
    b) False

41. A cardiologist has prescribed for a patient to get a digoxin injection. What volume of a 0.5 mg/2 mL digoxin injection will deliver the newly ordered dose of 0.25 mg?
    a) 1mL
    b) 0.5mL
    c) 2mL
    d) 4mL

42. Which of the following is found in the sulfonylurea classification?
    a) Glucotrol
    b) Minocin
    c) Relafen
    d) Aldactone

43. Diazepam is a _____ controlled substance.
    a) C II
    b) C III
    c) C IV
    d) C V

44. An elderly patient with advanced infection has been getting vancomycin 1750mg IVPB q8h. If this drug is stocked in 2g/10mL vials, what volume of medication additive should the technician be adding to each piggyback?
    a) 8.75mL
    b) 6.75mL
    c) 1.1mL
    d) 0.9mL

45. A patient has just been prescribed the drug verapamil. The physican has ordered a drug from which classification?
    a) NSAID
    b) Diuretic
    c) Antibacterial
    d) Calcium channel blocker

46. The _____ is located where the esophagus joins the stomach.
    a) pyloric sphincter
    b) cardiac sphincter
    c) gastric sphincter
    d) enteral sphincter

47. The drug Minocin works best when taken with dairy products for best absorption and less risk of stomach upset.
    a) True
    b) False

48. An injection is ordered at 50mg/kg/day in up 3 divided doses. If a patient taking this medication weighs 165lbs what will the strength of each dose be if given TID?
    a) 75mg
    b) 1250mg
    c) 37.5mg
    d) 150mg

49. Bile is produced by the gall bladder and stored in the liver until needed.
   a) True   b) False

50. Metoclopramide is classed as a(n) _____.
   a) Laxative   c) Anticholinergic/antispasmodic
   b) Proton pump inhibitor   d) GI stimulant

51. Antacids do not suppress gastric acid secretions like other GI meds do.
   a) True   b) False

52. In the duodenum, amylase begins to break down _____.
   a) proteins into amino acids   c) fats into micelles
   b) carbohydrates into simple sugars   d) electrolytes into simple salts

53. The generic name for Colace is docusate sodium.
   a) True   b) False

54. Relafen is known as a(n) _____.
   a) benzodiazepine   c) Antibacterial agent
   b) NSAID   d) Sulfonylurea

55. In the colon, the remaining contents of the gut can include _____.
   a) Dead cells   c) Undigestable roughage
   b) Water, other fluids and salts   d) All of these

56. Other than the location, the appendix has no direct connection to digestion or its processes.
   a) True   b) False

57. Antiflatulents are indicated to relieve _____ and most can be bought OTC.
   a) Diarrhea   c) Gas
   b) Constipation   d) Nausea

58. The brand or trade name for famotidine is _____.
   a) Pepcid   c) Prilosec
   b) Zantac   d) Prevacid

59. The colon is the same as the _____.
   a) Small intestine   b) Large intestine

60. Which of the following medications is not a proton pump inhibitor?
   a) Nexium   c) Pepcid
   b) Prevacid   d) Protonix

61. Friendly bacteria in the colon feed on the waste mixture in the colon and change it to feces.
   a) True
   b) False

62. A transplant patient has been ordered tacrolimus IV at 0.1mg/kg/day in continuous infusion. If the patient weighs 220 lbs, how many milligrams should be used as an additive?
   a) 100mg
   b) 1000mg
   c) 10mg
   d) 1mg

63. A 58 year old male weighing 209lbs has been prescribed Amphotericin injection. The recommended dosage is 4mg/kg/day. The once daily approach can be used for the entire amount or the dose can be given in a two equally divided injections. If BID dosing was chosen, what would be the proper amount per recommendations?
   a) 380mg
   b) 190mg
   c) 95mg
   d) 47.5mg

64. Stool softeners generally do not cause stimulation like laxatives do.
   a) True
   b) False

65. A patient has been suffering from flatulence as of late and his physician has recommended an over the counter product. Which is a probable recommendation?
   a) Imodium
   b) Mylicon
   c) Colace
   d) Maalox

66. The pyloric sphincter is located where the stomach joins the small intestine.
   a) True
   b) False

67. Levbid is classified as a(n) _____.
   a) Proton pump inhibitor
   b) H_2 antagonist
   c) Antispasmodic
   d) Antidiarrheal

68. Once the food mixture known as chime passed from the stomach into the small intestine, which substances can readily be absorbed without further breakdown by the gut?
   a) Water
   b) Fats
   c) Complex Carbohydrates
   d) Electrolytes
   e) Proteins
   f) Both a and d
   g) Both b and c
   h) All of these

69. In the ileum, fats, proteins and carbohydrates are all broken down where they can be absorbed by the body and used for energy.
   a) True
   b) False

70. Anticholinergic/antispasmodic medications act to _____ the motility in the GI tract.
   a) Stimulate
   b) Increase
   c) Decrease
   d) None of these

71. _____ are produced by friendly bacteria found in the colon.
   a) Enzymes
   b) Vitamins
   c) Both of these
   d) Neither of these

72. Most antacids require a prescription from a physician.
   a) True
   b) False

73. _____ promote bulk density in the bowel, slow down motility and help to diminish the loss of fluids.
   a) Antiflatulants
   b) Antidiarrheals
   c) Laxatives
   d) Stool softeners

74. Which of the following is not indicated to ease bowel movement?
   a) Lactulose
   b) Bisacodyl
   c) Loperamide
   d) Sennosides

75. A patient came to the pharmacy and purchased loperamide capsules. The patient is probably experiencing _____.
   a) Flatulence
   b) Constipation
   c) Nausea
   d) Diarrhea

76. The drug Lomotil is classed as a(n) _____.
   a) Anti-emetic
   b) Anti-diarrheal
   c) Laxative
   d) Antiflatulent

Match the following drugs to their generic names.

77. Calan SR   _____ a) doxycycline
78. Vibramycin   _____ b) glipizide
79. Biaxin   _____ c) clarithromycin
80. Synthroid   _____ d) verapamil
81. Minocin   _____ e) mupirocin
82. Compazine   _____ f) nabumetone
83. Relafen   _____ g) thyroid
84. Valium   _____ h) spironolactone
85. Glucotrol   _____ i) prochlorperazine
86. Bactroban   _____ j) levothyroxin
87. Armour Thyroid   _____ k) diazepam
88. Aldactone   _____ l) minocycline

Match the following drugs to their classifications.

89. Doxycycline   _____ a) calcium channel blocker

90. Verapamil   _____ b) thyroid hormone replacement

91. Thyroid   _____ c) sulfonylurea

92. Clarithromycin   _____ d) thyroid hormone replacement

93. diazepam   _____ e) topical antibacterial

94. Levothyroxine   _____ f) NSAID

95. Nabumetone   _____ g) tetracycline derivative antibacterial

96. Prochlorperazine   _____ h) macrolide antibacterial

97. Glipizide   _____ i) potassium sparing diuretic

98. Spironolactone   _____ j) antiemetic

99. Minocycline   _____ k) tetracycline derivative antibacterial

100. Mupirocin   _____ l) C IV benzodiazepine

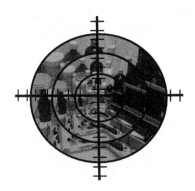

Mission 10
The Endrocrine System
Medications and Malfunctions

Mission Objectives

*To understand the basic anatomy and physiology of the endocrine system.

*To learn of the drug families used in treating endocrine disorders.

*To understand the pharmacology of drugs used in treating endocrine disorders.

*To gain baseline knowledge of twelve of the most popular drugs on the market.

*To review the principles of calculating flow rates for intravenous fluids including drops per minute, milliliters per hour, total volume and total run time

All body systems do not work individually, or on their own. Instead, they are completely dependent on each other for maintaining healthy bodily functions. Although, the nervous system is the ringleader of it all, there is another system that is not far behind in complexity and importance to the body. It is called the **endocrine system.**

Unlike other systems, which are primarily made up of like tissues, the endocrine system has many different parts with different functions. In fact, the organs of this awesome system are not directly connected with each other. The only thing that each of the glands or organs of this system has in common is the fact that they all produce **hormones**.

Each hormone is different and serves a different purpose to the body. Hormones assist in regulating and controlling some of the most important bodily functions. The organ that is affected by a specific hormone is called its **target organ**. Only that particular organ can receive that particular hormone, due to the fact that only the target organ's cells are designed to receive the chemical message that is in each specific hormone. It compares to a lock and key mechanism. The target organ would be the lock and the hormone would be the key that would trigger or open that lock to bring about a needed action or function.

There are three ways endocrine hormones can affect the body.

*   **Temporarily** the body might need a burst of energy, due to an emergency situation. Certain hormones produced in the adrenal glands trigger actions in the body that can help bring about added strength or resistance needed during such a time.

*   **Long term** needs could be recognized in such bodily activities as metabolism, which is a function that begins at birth and does not cease until death. This is something the body must do daily to produce and use energy. Hormones from the thyroid gland are responsible for this action.

*   **Short and long term** needs can be seen in the reproductive system. When we are young and not ready for reproduction, hormones are released at a minimum level. At puberty, the body goes through changes that bring about development of the organs and maintains a new level of hormones to keep the reproductive cycle functioning. As the body ages and reproduction is no longer needed, hormone levels are again reduced to a minimum operating level.

---

*   Pituitary
*   Adrenal,
*   Thyroid
*   Parathyroid
*   Pineal
*   Pancreas
*   Gonads
*   Thymus

There are eight individual glands in the endocrine system. The hypothalamus is not actually part of the endocrine system, but one of its functions is to control the pituitary gland. It is sometimes referred to as the mastermind of the endocrine system because it is the primary connection between the nervous and endocrine systems.

The **pituitary gland** is a pea-size gland situated under the lower rear of the brain. It produces hormones and its anterior and posterior lobes work separately.

The anterior lobe produces six of the eight pituitary hormones. The first of these is the **growth hormone (GH).** This regulates the way the body uses protein to make it grow. The next hormone, **adrenocorticotropic hormone (ACTH)**, stimulates the adrenal gland. Thyrotropic**,** or **thyroid-stimulating hormone (TSH)** helps in the function of another gland. It keeps the thyroid gland healthy and stimulates the production of thyroxine.

The two **gonadotropic** hormones act on the reproductive organs. The **follicle-stimulating hormone (FSH)** stimulates the ovaries to release an ovum, or egg. The **luteinizing hormone (LH)** stimulates the production of testosterone. **Prolactin** is another substance involved in regulating reproduction organs. It stimulates the mammary glands in a pregnant woman's breast to develop and produce milk needed to feed and nourish an infant.

The posterior lobe of the pituitary gland produces two hormones. **Oxytocin** causes the muscles in a woman's uterus to contract during labor and delivery. It also allows contraction of the muscles in a mother's breast to allow milk to flow into a nursing infant's mouth. **Antidiuretic Hormone (ADH)** regulates urine output to keep the level of water in the body controlled. ADH also stimulates contraction of the smooth muscle in arterial tissue; therefore it increases the blood pressure when needed.

The pair of **adrenal glands** is situated above the kidneys. The inner area, called the adrenal medulla, produces totally different hormones than the outer area, known as the adrenal cortex.

The **adrenal medulla** produces **adrenaline (epinephrine)** and **noradrenaline (norepinephrine).** Adrenaline causes an increase in heart rate and blood sugar. It also increases the body's alertness during emergency or stressful situations. Noradrenaline increases blood pressure.

The hormones produced by the **adrenal cortex** are called **corticosteroids**. The two main ones are cortisol and aldosterone. **Cortisol** gets produced and released when the body is stressed. The pituitary gland sends ACTH to the adrenal glands to trigger this production. **Aldosterone**, helps the intestines, kidneys and sweat glands to regulate the water and salt levels in the body.

The **thyroid gland** is located at the front of the neck. It is a butterfly shaped organ with two lobes (one on each side of the trachea) that are connected by a bridge of tissue called the isthmus. The thyroid releases the hormones it produces, when it is stimulated by the thyrotropic hormone (TSH) from the pituitary gland. **Thyroxine** brings about or stimulates metabolism while **calcitonin** sends calcium to the bones where it is needed for growth, development and maintenance of strong bones.

There are four **parathyroid glands** situated against the surface of the thyroid gland. These glands produce **parahormone**. This substance helps the body to take in and use calcium and phosphate salts. Parahormone also acts with calcitonin to regulate calcium levels in the body.

The **pineal gland** is found in the center of the brain. It secretes the hormone, **melatonin**. This hormone is believed to help regulate the wake-sleep cycle. Research tells that upsets in the secretion of melatonin are responsible for the jet lag we feel when we have had to travel by air for a long period of time.

The **pancreas** is the body's second largest gland. Its primary function is to produce the hormone **insulin**. When the body's sugar level gets to a certain amount, insulin assists the cells in absorbing the glucose. The pancreas also stops the liver from sending excess glucose to the blood and helps the muscles store glycogen for future use. If the pancreas fails to produce enough insulin, all of these important sugar-absorbing functions get disrupted and the disease known as diabetes is the result.

The shortage of insulin causes a high blood glucose level because the sugar is unable to be absorbed without insulin. The cells become starved for energy, as well as the chemical balance getting "off balance" and upset. Delicate tissues could become damaged including eyes, skin, nerves, liver and kidneys.

The **gonads** are the reproductive glands. These are the only glands that differ between males and females. Males have **testes** and females have **ovaries**. These glands act when they are stimulated by the gonadotropic hormone from the pituitary gland.

The testes major function is to produce sperm. It also releases **testosterone**. The ovaries major function is to produce ova, or eggs, but they also release the hormones, **estrogen** and **progesterone**. The hormones produced by the reproductive glands are responsible for the characteristics of gender. These include, but are not limited to deeper voices, facial and pubic hair and development of external reproductive organs in the male. In the female, wider pelvic bones, pubic hair and breast development is noticed. These hormones also help to control reproduction, release of ova, and development of sperm cells and events of conception.

Though some sources do not recognize the **thymus gland** as part of the endocrine system, it is believed to produce **thymosins**, which are hormones, and that brings the connection to the endocrine system for most of the sources available. The thymus is located in the upper chest and parts of its exact role are still a mystery. It is believed to be vital to the development of antibodies, especially T cells, which help with the body's immune system. The two hormones that the thymus releases regulate the maturation of T cells. After puberty, the thymus gets smaller and smaller with time and eventually ceases to function at all.

The **hypothalamus** is not part of the endocrine system, but it is the mastermind behind the production and the release of hormones from the glands. It has the ability to monitor the blood levels of hormones and send chemical signals to the hormone producing glands to either raise or lower the levels. All in all, you can see why the endocrine system is so complex and important to normal bodily functions.

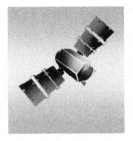

Recon Mission 10:

There are so many different diseases that can be associated with the endocrine system. With this mission's reconnaissance you are encouraged to search the Internet for information on various diseases and disorders of the endocrine system. Also seek out anatomical diagrams of the endocrine system so that each area becomes more familiar to you now that a review of the functionality has been completed. Many websites offer interactive diagrams which allow you to label and maneuver them.

Write down as many of the conditions as you can find with a brief description of each one. As you continue on this mission, some medications may be discussed that are used primarily to treat diseases and disorders that you have read about and familiarized yourself with. As a guide only, the following bulleted points could be used as keywords in your search. Each keyword suggested below may have multiple possible inclusions for your review. You are encouraged to devote plenty of time to this activity.

* Endocrine System diseases and disorders
* Endocrine illnesses
* Interactive diagrams of the Endocrine System

Medications for Malfunctions

There are many drug classes that affect the Endocrine system. Here you will learn of the basic classes and their pharmacological actions on the body. Take into consideration that true pharmacology goes much deeper than you will learn in this preparatory course, but you should obtain enough information to understand the basic actions on the body for these medications.

Estrogens are components in combination contraceptives or as hormone replacement therapy in postmenopausal women. They affect the release of pituitary gonadotropic hormone, cause capillary dilatation, fluid retention, protein anabolism, increase water content of cervical mucous and inhibit ovulation.

* Estrace - Estradiol
* Ogen - Estropipate
* Premarin - Conjugated estrogens

Progestins increase endometrial receptivity necessary for implantation for embryo. Once an embryo is implanted progestins act to maintain the pregnancy. The drugs in this family are used in conditions where endometrial activity is the problem such as abnormal bleeding or endometriosis. In patients undergoing estrogen replacement therapy, the progestins are indicated to reduce incidence of emdometrial hyperplasia.

> Progestins are beneficial only to those patients with an intact uterus. With no uterus, a patient would have no need to take a drug in this class.

* Provera - Medroxyprogesterone
* Prometrium – Progesterone

There are some combination medications that contain both estrogens and progestins to make this much easier for post menopausal patients.
* Prempro – conjugated estrogens / medroxyprogesterone
* Femhrt & Activella - estradiol/norethindrone

Contraceptives are indicated for the prevention of pregnancy. They inhibit ovulation by suppression of gonadotropic hormones FSH and LH. They also cause alterations in the genital tract, cervical mucous and endometrium. Most contraceptives contain a combination of both estrogens such as estradiol and progestins such as norethindrone. Though they are available in quarterly injectable, weekly patch and even a permanently placed device of different sorts, the "pill" is still the most common form of birth control for those patients who are using contraceptive methods other than permanent sterilization.

Traditionally, oral contraceptives include 3 weeks of active hormone tablets and 1 week of placebo or inert tablets. During the week of inert tablets, they are there primarily as a reminder to "take the pill" daily and the monthly cycle occurs.

There are so many different variations of these oral birth control pills so their generic names and strengths of ingredients have been intentionally omitted. Some versions offer extended day packs with up to 3 months of active hormone tablets before allowing a "down time" of hormonal dosing to allow for a normal menstrual cycle.

* Ovral
* Lo-Ovral
* Ortho-Cept
* Ortho-Tri-Cylen
* Triphasil
* LoEstrin FE 24
* Seasonale

Ovulations stimulants are used to treat ovulatory failure. They induce ovulation by sending false signals to the pituitary and hypothalamus that the estrogen levels are low. This brings about increased secretion of FSH, LH and gonadotropic hormones resulting in ovarian stimulation.

* Clomid – Clomiphene Citrate

Uterine-activants such as oxytocin are given during labor to induce or improve contractions. It can also be given post-partum to speed up delivery of placenta ad help control intra-uterine bleeding.

* Pitocin – Oxytocin

On the other hand, **uterine relaxants** are given during pre-term labor to stop or post-pone uterine contractions. These drugs work as a Beta$_2$ receptor agonist, which exerts preferential effect on Beta$_2$ adrenergic receptors, particularly those found in uterine smooth muscle.

* Yutopar – Ritodrine

First generation **androgens** are used for hormone replacement therapy in males due to testicular failure, impotence and other problems. These androgens are taken regularly to "replace" hormones not being naturally produced. In addition to oral dosage forms, these androgens also are available in injectable and topical forms.

* Halotestin – Fluoxymesterone
* Android – Methyltestosterone
* Androgel – Testosterone topical

In the newer age of HRT for male patients, **exogenous androgen therapy** with agents indicated for erectile dysfunction (ED) can be administered on an as desired basis.

* Viagra – Sildenafil
* Cialis – Tadalafil
* Levitra - Vardenafil

Glucocorticoids are adrenocortical steroids. They cause profound and varied metabolic effects. Also they modify the body's immune responses to diverse stimuli. In essence, these agents help the body to heal faster or resist rejection of a healing process.

* Decadron – Dexamethasone
* Medrol – Methylprednisolone
* Deltasone – Prednisone
* Pediapred - Prednisolone

Thyroid hormones are given for hormone replacement in patients who suffer from hypothyroidism. Their mechanism of action is not completely understood.

* Armour Thyroid – Thyroid
* Synthroid – Levothyroxine

Anti-Thyroid agents are given to treat a condition known as hyperthyroidism which is much less common than the earlier mentioned thyroid condition. These medications inhibit the synthesis of thyroid hormone.

* Tapazole – Methimazole
* PTU – Propylthiouracil

Anti-Gout agents such as allopurinol are given to reduce and maintain the production of uric acid. Other gout agents such as Colchicine are indicated for acute attacks of gout to relieve pain.

* Zyloprim – Allopurinol
* Colchicine

Insulin is an **antidiabetic agent** used in treatment of Types 1 & 2 diabetes mellitus, hyperkalemia, and ketoacidosis. It replaces the insulin that cannot or is not being produced by the beta cells in the pancreas.

Regular insulin is rapid acting with a faster peak and shorter duration. NPH insulin is intermediate acting with about the same peak time but with a longer duration. 70/30 insulin is a combination of both NPH (70%) and regular (30%) insulins. There are some long acting insulins that are used more by those patients who are in better control of their medical condition.

Today's technologies have allowed diabetic patients more opportunities and options with their dependence on injectable insulin. There are different insulin pumps and new fangled glucometers that help them to take better care of themselves. Typically a person using insulin should not change dosages or brands unless instructed to do so by a physician. With so many variations of insulin available, the generic names have been intentionally omitted.

* Novolin brands of NPH, Regular and 70/30
* Novolog and Novolog Mix 75/25
* Humulin brands of NPH, Regular and 70/30
* Lantus and Levemir

Other antidiabetic agents called **sulfonylureas** are used in conjunction with diet and exercise to lower blood glucose levels in patients with Type 2 diabetes. They bind to plasma membrane of beta cells in the pancreatic islets and ultimately increase insulin secretion.

* Diabenese – Chlorpropamide 1st generation
* Tolinase   - Tolazamide
* Orinase   - Tolbutamide

* Glucotrol   – Glipizide 2nd generation
* Micronase – Glyburide

Alpha Glucosidase Inhibitors do not enhance insulin secretion. Instead, they work by a reversible inhibition of the pancreatic enzyme, alpha-amylase. In diabetic patients, this enzyme inhibition will slow glucose absorption and enhance glycemic control.

* Precose – Acarbose

Biguanides are also used in treatment of type 2 when diet alone won't work.. They improve glucose tolerance by lowering both basal and post-prandial (after mealtime) plasma glucose. Its mechanism of action includes decreased hepatic glucose production, decreased intestinal absorption and improvement of insulin sensitivity.

* Glucophage – Metformin

Still other agents such as Actos increase insulin sensitivity. These meds are called **Thiazolidinediones** and they do not increase insulin secretion, only its sensitivity.

* Actos – Pioglitazone

Many of these medications that are in different classes are given together. Although the ultimate goal for all diabetic medications is to get the blood glucose level under control, most of the different meds have different mechanisms of action and will complement each other. Taking multiple medications for the same condition is not uncommon in diabetic patients. However, duplicate therapy – meaning two drugs from the same classification (ie two sulfonylureas) are not necessary.

A condition called hypoglycemia occurs when the blood glucose level gets too low. Glucose elevating agents like Glucagon injection or Glutose gel can be given to raise the glucose level.

Antidotes

Antidotes or detoxification agents are used to counteract another substance's action. Though these may not seem or be endocrinal, they may have various metabolic actions which produce results. Listed in the table below are these substances, their generic names and the toxin or substance that will be reversed. Sometimes an emetic such as ipecac is given in drug overdosage and certain poisonings where vomiting is needed. However, on occasion, a substance may cause more damage with vomiting. A charcoal substance helps to neutralize some poisonings and speed up their elimination in these situations.

Brand Name	Generic Name	Indication
Desferal	Deferoxamine	Iron overload
Calcium EDTA	Edetate Calcium Disodium (EDTA)	Lead poisoning
Sodium Thiosulfate	n/a	Cyanide poisoning
Narcan	Naloxone	Opiate overdose
Romazicon	Flumazenil	Benzodiazepine sedation
Antizol	Fomepizole	Ethylene glycol (antifreeze) or methanol poisoning
Digibind Digifab	Digoxin immune FAB	Digoxin overload
Mucomyst	Acetylcisteine	Acetaminophen overdose
Ipecac	Ipecac syrup	Accidental poisonings
Actidose CharcoAid	Activated charcoal	Accidental poisonings

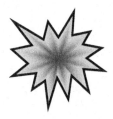

Math Blaster

For the Mission 10 Math Blaster, feel free to review the explanations in Mission 5 for the pharmacy calculations. In the mission 10 debriefing, you will be revisiting the skills learned in the earlier Mission.

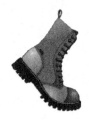

Drill Practice

For this mission's drill practice, rework those questions found in Mission 5 drill practice. In the Mission 10 debriefing, you will be checking to see how well you remember those skills.

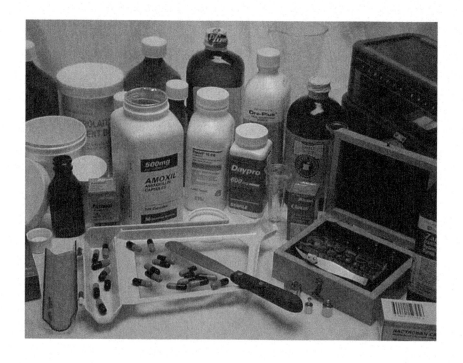

Drug Training Chapter Ten

Brand Name	Generic Name	Drug Classification	Primary Indication	Side effects, Warnings, Other
Inderal	Propranolol	Beta-adrenergic Receptor Blocker	Hypertension	Bradycardia, hypotension, parasthesia, fatigue, light-headedness, GI upset
Antivert	Meclizine	Anti-histamine	Motion sickness, Vertigo	Drowsiness, Dry Mouth
Rozerem	Ramelteon	Hypnotic	Insomnia characterized by difficulty with sleep onset	Somnolence, dizziness, nausea, fatigue, headache, insomnia
Paxil	Paroxetine	Selective Serotonin Reuptake Inhibitor (SSRI)	Major Depressive Disorder, Obsessive-Compulsive Disorder, Panic or Anxiety Disorder	May increase risk of suicidal thinking and behavior (suicidality) in children, adolescents, and young adults; Asthenia, sweating, nausea, decreased appetite, somnolence, dizziness, insomnia, tremor, nervousness, ejaculatory disturbance
Desyrel	Trazodone	antidepressant	Depression	May increase the risk of suicidal thinking and behavior children, adolescents and young adults. Drowsiness, dizziness, nervousness, dry mouth, nausea and vomiting,
Oxycontin	Oxycodone	CII Opioid Analgesic	Moderate to severe pain	constipation, nausea, somnolence, dizziness, vomiting, pruritus, headache, dry mouth, sweating, and asthenia
Avapro	Irbesartan	Angiotensen II Receptor Blocker (ARB)	Hypertension	avoid during pregnancy; may cause diarrhea, dyspepsia, heartburn, fatigue
Voltaren	Diclofenac sodium	Non-Steroidal Anti-inflammatory Drug (NSAID)	Osteoarthritis, Rheumatoid Arthritis, Spondylitis	May increase risk of cardiovascular thrombotic events abdominal pain, GI upset and bleeding, anemia, dizziness, edema, elevated liver enzymes, headaches, rash

Brand Name	Generic Name	Drug Classification	Primary Indication	Side effects, Warnings, Other
Accupril	Quinapril	ACE inhibitor	Hypertension	Headache, Dizziness, Asthenia
Flagyl	Metronidazole	Antiprotozoal Antibacterial	treatment of symptomatic trichomoniasis in females and males when the presence of thetrichomonad has been confirmed by lab	Note: Alcohol should be avoided, GI upset, headache, mertallic taste, dizziness
Catapres	Clonidine	Centrally acting alpha-agonist	Hypertension	Dry mouth, dizziness, drowsiness, sedtion, constipation
Adalat CC, Procardia XL	Nifedipine	Calcium Channel Blocker	Hypertension	Avoid grapefruit juice; may cause headache, peripheral edema, paresthesia, dizziness, impotence

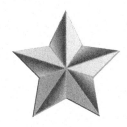

Mission 10 Debriefing

Answer the following questions in assessment of the lessons learned in Mission 10. For best results, repeat the exercise until no questions are missed then move on to the next mission.

1. Each of the glands in the endocrine system produces _____.
   a) antibodies
   b) blood cells
   c) enzymes
   d) hormones

2. Oxycodone is a _____ opioid analgesic indicated for moderate to severe pain.
   a) C II
   b) C III
   c) C IV
   d) C V

3. The testes produce and release estrogens.
   a) True
   b) False

4. The parathyroid glands produce _____.
   a) thyroxine
   b) calcitonin
   c) parahormone
   d) all of these

5. An i.v. infusion order is written for 1000mL of D5LR to run over 10 hours. The set you have will deliver 20gtts/mL. What should the flow rate be in gtts/min?
   a) 25gtts/min
   b) 33gtts/min
   c) 66gtts/min
   d) 100gtts/min

6. The follicle stimulating hormone (FSH) stimulates the _____.
   a) Thyroid gland to produce thyroxine
   b) Thyroid gland to produce calcitonin
   c) Ovaries to release ovum
   d) Testes to produce testosterone

7. Adrenaline causes an increase in _____.
   a) heart rate
   b) blood pressure
   c) blood sugar
   d) all of these
   e) both a and b
   f) both a and c

8. Estrogen and progesterone are produced by the pineal gland.
    a) True   b) False

9. Which of the following medications is indicated for hypertension?
    a) Adalat CC   c) Catapres
    b) Accupril   d) All of these

10. Melatonin sends calcium to the bones where it is needed for growth, development and maintenance of strong bones.
    a) True   b) False

11. Metformin is classed as a(n) _____.
    a) sulfonylurea   c) biguanide
    b) alpha glucosidase inhibitor   d) thiazolidinedione

12. _____ are used in patients with conditions involving trouble with endometrial activity such as abnormal bleeding or endometriosis.
    a) Estrogens   c) Progestins
    b) Androids   d) None of these

13. The thyroid gland is stimulated by thyrotropic hormone produced by the pituitary gland.
    a) True   b) False

14. If 1500mL of Lactated Ringers solution is to be given over 12 hours. Determine the mL/hr.
    a) 31mL/hr   c) 83mL/hr
    b) 52mL/hr   d) 125mL/hr

15. Thymosins, hormones produced by the thymus gland, are believed to be vital to the production of antibodies which help the body's immune system to function.
    a) True   b) False

16. The _____ gland's primary function is to produce the hormone insulin.
    a) pituitary   c) pineal
    b) pancreas   d) none of these

17. Which of the following pairs of medications increase the risk of suicidal thinking in young adults, children and adolescents?
    a) Inderal and Avapro   c) Voltaren and Oxycontin
    b) Desyrel and Paxil   d) Catapres and Accupril

18. Antidiuretic Hormone regulates urine output to keep the level of _____ controlled.
    a) Electrolytes
    c) Adrenaline
    b) Salts
    d) Water

19. A medication called _____ is indicated for pain with acute gout attacks.
    a) methimazole
    c) colchicine
    b) allopurinol
    d) levothyroxine

20. Romazicon is given to reverse _____ levels.
    a) opioid
    c) lead
    b) iron
    d) benzodiazepine

21. Thiazolidinediones increase insulin sensitivity not insulin secretion.
    a) True
    b) False

22. The drug _____ is indicated to increase insulin sensitivity in diabetics.
    a) Synthroid
    c) Zyloprim
    b) Actos
    d) Ogen

23. Deferoxamine is indicated for cyanide poisoning.
    a) True
    b) False

24. What is the total volume that will be needed if D5W is to run at 70mL/hr for 24 hours?
    a) 1680mL
    c) 1920mL
    b) 2916mL
    d) 1460mL

25. Which of the drugs is not an estrogen?
    a) Premarin
    d) All of these are estrogens
    b) Provera
    e) All of these are not estrogens
    c) Prometrium
    f) Both b and c are not

26. The adrenal medulla produces _____.
    a) Adrenaline
    c) Both a and b
    b) Noradrenaline
    d) Neither a nor b

27. A shortage in insulin production would result in an _____ blood glucose level.
    a) Increased
    c) Neither as insulin does not affect
    b) Decreased
       blood glucose.

28. The drug Rozerem is used for treating _____.
    a) depression
    b) insomnia
    c) pain
    d) neuropathy

29. The gonads are the only glands that differ between males and females.
    a) True
    b) False

30. An i.v. infusion order is written for 1000mL of Lactated Ringers to run over 16 hours. What should the flow rate be in mL/hr?
    a) 21mL/hr
    b) 56mL/hr
    c) 63mL/hr
    d) 83mL/hr

31. Estrogens are found in contraceptives and traditional hormone replacement therapies.
    a) True
    b) False

32. In which of the following ways can the endocrine system affect the body as a whole?
    a) Temporarily with a surge of hormones produced and released.
    b) Long term with a continuous hormonal activity produced and released.
    c) Both short and long term with hormones ranging from minimum to maximum levels to yield certain functions of the body for various periods of time.
    d) All of these are ways the endocrine system can function and affect the body.

33. "The pill" is still the most common form of birth control without permanent sterilization.
    a) True
    b) False

34. Diclofenac may increase the risk of _____.
    a) suicidal thinking
    b) tendonitis
    c) alopecia
    d) cardiovascular events

35. Thyroxine stimulates metabolism function.
    a) True
    b) False

36. _____ would be given during labor to induce or improve contractions.
    a) Pitocin
    b) Yutopar
    c) Clomid
    d) None of these

37. How many 500mL bags will be needed if a patient receives D5W at 50mL/hr for 12 hours?
    a) 1 bag
    b) 2 bags
    c) 3 bags
    d) 4 bags

38. _____ helps the intestines, kidneys and sweat glands to regulate water and salt levels in the body.
   a) Aldosterone
   b) Noradrenaline
   c) Oxytocin
   d) Calcitonin

39. The drug Paxil is in what classification of antidepressants?
   a) Tricyclics
   b) SNRIs
   c) SSRIs
   d) It is not an antidepressant

40. Contraceptives are indicated for pregnancy prevention.
   a) True
   b) False

41. The hormone which stimulates or triggers the adrenal gland is _____.
   a) cortisol
   b) adrenocorticotropic
   c) adrenaline
   d) aldosterone

42. An i.v. infusion order is written for 1000mL of $D_5W/0.225\%NS$ to run over 14 hours. The set you have will deliver 20gtts/mL. What should the flow rate be in mL/hr?
   a) 24mL/hr
   b) 48mL/hr
   c) 71mL/hr
   d) 125mL/hr

43. A patient has recently been written a prescription for a calcium channel blocker. Which of the drugs below may have been prescribed?
   a) Accupril
   b) Procardia XL
   c) Catapres
   d) Avapro

44. Growth hormone (GH) regulates how the body uses sugars to make it grow.
   a) True
   b) False

45. What is the total volume that will be needed if D5LR is to run at 125mL/hr for 10 hours?
   a) 1000mL
   b) 1250mL
   c) 1500mL
   d) 1750mL

46. 1000mL of dextrose solution is to be given over 8 hours. Determine the number of gtts/min if the set you're using delivers 10gtts/mL.
   a) 125gtts/min
   b) 84gtts/min
   c) 63gtts/min
   d) 21gtts/min

47. Nifedipine is an ACE inhibitor indicated for treatment of hypertension.
   a) True
   b) False

48. The _____ has the ability to monitor blood levels of hormones and signal hormone producing glands to raise or lower production levels.
   a) Thalamus
   b) Medulla oblongata
   c) Hypothalamus
   d) Cerebellum

49. Which of the following medications could be administered in case of accidental poisoning where vomiting is not recommended?
   a) Ipecac syrup
   b) Activated charcoal
   c) Either a or b
   d) Neither a nor b

50. What is the flow rate in gtts/min if 1000mL of D5NS is to be given over 12 hours and the set delivers 15gtts/mL?
   a) 21gtts/min
   b) 28gtts/min
   c) 56gtts/min
   d) 83gtts/min

51. The adrenal cortex produces _____.
   a) Adrenaline and noradrenaline
   b) Cortisol and aldosterone
   c) Thyroxine and calcitonin
   d) Melatonin and prolactin

52. When a patient is taking metronidazole, which of the substances below should be avoided due to a interaction?
   a) Grapefruit juice
   b) Dairy products
   c) Antacids
   d) Alcohol products

53. Allopurinol is indicated to reduce/maintain the production of uric acid in gout patients.
   a) True
   b) False

54. _____ stimulates the mammary glands in the breast to develop and produce milk to feed and nourish an infant.
   a) Adrenaline
   b) Prolactin
   c) Cortisol
   d) Oxytocin

55. How many 1L bags will be needed if a patient is getting Half Normal Saline continuous infusion at a rate of 100mL/hr for 14 hours?
   a) 1 bag
   b) 2 bags
   c) 3 bags
   d) 4 bags

56. The pineal gland produces _____.
   a) cortisol
   b) thyroxine
   c) oxytocin
   d) melatonin

57. Paroxetine and trazodone are indicated to treat _____.
    a) Osteoarthritis
    c) Hypertension
    b) Depression
    d) Pain

58. Which of the following helps the body take in and use calcium and phosphate salts?
    a) Parahormone
    c) Thyroxine
    b) Calcitonin
    d) None of these

59. Which of the following medications would be administered to a patient with acetaminophen overdose?
    a) Desferal
    c) Mucomyst
    b) Narcan
    d) Actidose

60. What is the flow rate in mL/hr if 1000mL of D_5W is to be given over 6 hours and the set delivers 20gtts/mL?
    a) 42mL/hr
    c) 111mL/hr
    b) 56mL/hr
    d) 167mL/hr

61. The drug Prometrium is used in estrogen replacement therapy.
    a) True
    b) False

62. _____ causes the muscles in a woman's uterus to contract during labor.
    a) Prolactin
    c) Adrenaline
    b) Oxytocin
    d) Noradrenaline

63. Calcitonin is responsible for _____.
    a) helping the body take in and use calcium and phosphate salts.
    b) sending calcium to the bones for growth, development and maintenance.
    c) stimulating metabolism function.
    d) producing and distributing insulin.

64. Sodium thiosulfate should be administered if a patient is found with digoxin overload.
    a) True
    b) False

65. Medications from which of the following pairs would be indicated for patients suffering from hyperthyroidism?
    a) Glyburide or Metformin
    c) Thyroid or Levothyroxine
    b) Methimazole or Propylthiouracil
    d) Allopurinol or Colchicine

66. Luteinizing Hormone (LH) stimulates the production of testosterone.
    a) True
    b) False

67. Which of these drugs is indicated to lower blood pressure?
    a) Avapro
    b) Inderal
    c) Both a and b
    d) Neither a nor b

68. Both prednisone and dexamethasone are glucocorticoids.
    a) True
    b) False

69. Naloxone reverses an overload of what substance in the blood?
    a) Digoxin
    b) Opioids
    c) Cyanide
    d) Iron

70. The organ affected by a specific hormone is that hormone's target organ.
    a) True
    b) False

71. An i.v. infusion order is written for 1000mL of $D_5W/0.45\%NS$ to run over 8 hours. The set you have will deliver 15gtts/mL. What should the flow rate be in gtts/min?
    a) 31gtts/min
    b) 56gtts/min
    c) 83gtts/min
    d) 125gtts/min

72. Which of the following pairs of medications are sulfonylurea drugs?
    a) Glucophage and pioglitazone
    b) Acarbose and glucophage
    c) Glipizide and glyburide
    d) Methimazole and propylthiouracil

73. Thyroid stimulating hormone is released from the _____ gland.
    a) Thyroid
    b) Adrenal
    c) Parathyroid
    d) Pituitary

74. Biguanides such as Glucophage have which of the following pharmacologic actions?
    a) Decreased intestinal absorption of glucose
    b) Decreased hepatic production of glucose for storage
    c) Improvement of insulin sensitivity
    d) All of these

75. Grapefruit juice should be avoided when taking nifedipine.
    a) True
    b) False

76. Which of the following is not an exogenous androgen therapy medication?
    a) Androgel
    b) Viagra
    c) Levitra
    d) Cialis

242

Match the following drugs to their generic names.

77. Inderal   _____ a) nifedipine
78. Voltaren   _____ b) metronidazole
79. Catapres   _____ c) diclofenac sodium
80. Accupril   _____ d) oxycodone
81. Desyrel   _____ e) paroxetine
82. Avapro   _____ f) meclizine
83. Flagyl   _____ g) propranolol
84. Procardia XL   _____ h) clonidine
85. Paxil   _____ i) quinapril
86. Antivert   _____ j) irbesartan
87. Rozerem   _____ k) trazodone
88. Oxycontin   _____ l) ramelteon

Match the following drugs to their classifications.

89. Propranolol   _____ a) calcium channel blocker
90. Ramelteon   _____ b) antidepressant
91. Trazodone   _____ c) centrally acting alpha-agonist
92. Irbesartan   _____ d) hypnotic
93. Quinapril   _____ e) antiprotozoal antibacterial
94. Clonidine   _____ f) NSAID
95. Nifedipine   _____ g) C II opioid analgesic
96. Metronidazole   _____ h) SSRI
97. Diclofenac Sodium   _____ i) antihistamine
98. Oxycodone   _____ j) beta blocker
99. Paroxetine   _____ k) ACE inhibitor
100. Meclizine   _____ l) angiotensin II receptor blocker (ARB)

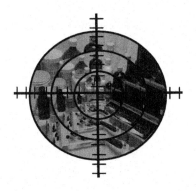

Mission 11
The Cardiovascular System
Medications and Malfunctions

Mission Objectives

*To understand the basic anatomy and physiology of the cardiovascular system and its components.

*To become familiar with the path that blood travels through the body.

*To learn of the drug families used in treating cardiovascular disorders.

*To understand the pharmacology of drugs used in treating cardiovascular disorders.

*To gain baseline knowledge of twelve of the most popular drugs on the market.

*To review calculations used in compounding including allegations and concentrations and dilutions.

This body system is as awesome in itself as the other systems we've studied thus far. It is made up of the heart, arteries, veins and capillaries. It is a closed system consisting of approximately 90,000 miles of blood vessel through which the heart pumps around 5,000 to 6,000 quarts of blood in a single day. The **cardiovascular system** is the major transportation system for the body. It is how nutrients and oxygen are carried to the tissues, as well as, how wastes and toxins are carried to those body parts which filter the blood.

The **heart** is a fist-sized organ composed of strong muscle. This muscle contracting and relaxing is what pushes the blood through the blood vessels and eventually back to the heart

The **vena cava** brings the blood from the body back into the heart. It enters the heart at the **right atrium**. The blood is then forced into the **right ventricle** through the **tricuspid valve**. As it leaves the right ventricle through the **pulmonary valve** it travels to the lungs by way of the pulmonary artery. In the lungs, blood is reoxygenated and sent back to the heart through the **pulmonary vein**. The blood reenters the heart at the **left atrium**. It then goes through the **mitral valve** into the **left ventricle**. After leaving the left ventricle, blood is pumped through the **aortic valve** into the **aortic arch** and **aorta**. Now the blood is headed out to the body tissues to carry fresh oxygen.

Blood travels first through the aorta, the largest artery, which is approximately one inch in diameter. It receives blood from the heart at a rate of about 16 inches per second. As the blood moves further away from the heart the aorta divides into other smaller main **arteries** which branch off into even smaller arteries, and eventually even smaller arteries called **arterioles**. Artery walls are very tough and muscular and need to be in order to withstand the vigorous pressure that is placed on them with each contraction of the heart. These arterial vessel structures vary in size from one-sixth to one-fourth of an inch in diameter. They can contract or expand depending on the tissues' need for blood. Such activity or change in diameter is regulated by the autonomic nervous system.

The arterioles branch into even tinier vessels called **capillaries**. These capillaries are smaller and supersede both veins and arteries in number. Many cells will pass through capillary tissues in single file because the entire diameter is only about $1/3500$ of an inch wide and just slightly larger than a red blood cell. Here in the capillaries is where the **oxygen exchange** for the tissues takes place. Oxygen and nutrients are given to the tissues and waste and carbon dioxide are given back to the capillaries. The blood is filtered for waste products as it passes through the kidneys. The capillaries begin the return of blood back to the heart.

The pulmonary artery is the only artery that carries blood low in oxygen and likewise, the pulmonary vein is the only vein that carries fresh oxygenated . . .

The capillaries eventually connect with the **venules** and then larger **veins**. The walls of veins are thinner and much more flexible than those of arteries. As the blood nears the end of its journey back to the heart the pressure in the veins is weak and as a result the blood flows much slower and more smoothly. Many larger veins, especially those in the legs, have one-way valves that prevent the backflow of blood due to gravity. The larger veins all dump into either the **superior** (upper) or **inferior** (lower) vena cava finally connect with the main **vena cava**, which empties directly into the heart.

Though the heart is responsible for forcing the blood transportation through the body, it too, needs a fresh blood supply in order to maintain its normal function. The heart muscle, often referred to as the **myocardium**, is fed this fresh blood supply from its own network of right and left **coronary arteries** directly branching from the aorta. As the blood flows through coronary arteries, into capillaries and eventually into coronary veins, this blood is deposited into the larger **coronary sinus vein** which empties its contents directly into the right atrium and the process continues on repeatedly.

The heart only stops for a moment in between beats. The contraction phase is called **systole**. The brief moment of relaxation is called a **diastole**. Blood pressure is measured at the two points of contraction and relaxation by a device known as a **sphygmomanometer**. This device will render systolic and diastolic blood pressure respectively. For instance, a blood pressure reading that is 120/80 has a systolic reading of 120 and a diastolic reading of 80.

Another component of the cardiovascular system is the vehicle by which nutrients and oxygen are transported to the body's cells. **Blood** is also the way of transport for carbon dioxide and wastes to be expelled from those cells. It totals about 11 pints and makes up approximately one-twelfth of the average adult's body weight.

Everyone has one of four **blood types** or groups. The types are differed by the **antigens** (markers) on the red blood cells. The different types also carry different **antibodies** in their plasma. If blood types are not matched with the proper donor/patient, clumping can occur which will upset the normal flow of blood and can be detrimental to the receiving patient. Therefore, blood types must be cross matched and medical staff members are diligent in their efforts to make sure that the proper blood type is given during a transfusion. The types are as follows.

* Type A – contains A antigens with B antibodies in the plasma.
* Type B – contains B antigens with A antibodies in the plasma.
* Type AB – contains both A and B antigens with neither A nor B antibodies in the plasma.
* Type O – contains neither A nor B antigens but contains both A and B antibodies in the plasma.

Blood is suspension-like in nature meaning that the various parts of the whole can be separated. It is composed of four main parts. About 55% of blood is plasma. This **plasma** is mostly water but it also contains nutrients, inorganic materials, proteins, antibodies and hormones. The other 45% of blood is composed of cells. There are three kinds of blood cells: Red blood cells, white blood cells and platelets.

The **red blood cells**, often called **erythrocytes**, carry oxygen to the cells and carry off wastes and carbon dioxide. They have a lifespan of about three or four months and then are replaced by new ones produced by bone marrow. The **white blood cells**, or **leukocytes**, protect the body from harmful toxic organisms by consuming and destroying them. Though the white blood cells are outnumbered by red blood cells normally at about 700 to 1, an infection can cause the white count to double within just a few short hours. The other type of cells found in the blood is **platelets**. These cells assist in blood clotting also called coagulation.

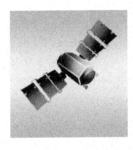

Recon Mission 11:

There are so many different diseases that can be associated with the cardiovascular system. With this mission's reconnaissance you are encouraged to search the Internet for information on various diseases and disorders of the cardiovascular system. Also seek out anatomical diagrams of the cardiovascular system so that each area becomes more familiar to you now that a review of the functionality has been completed. Many websites offer interactive diagrams which allow you to label and maneuver them.

Write down as many of the conditions as you can find with a brief description of each one. As you continue on this mission, some medications may be discussed that are used primarily to treat diseases and disorders that you have read about and familiarized yourself with. As a guide only, the following bulleted points could be used as keywords in your search. Each keyword suggested below may have multiple possible inclusions for your review. You are encouraged to devote plenty of time to this activity.

* Cardiovascular System diseases and disorders
* Circulatory illnesses
* Interactive diagrams of the Cardiovascular System

Medications for Malfunctions

There are many drug classes that affect the Cardiovascular system. Here you will learn of the basic classes and their pharmacological actions on the body. Take into consideration that true pharmacology goes much deeper than you will learn in this preparatory course, but you should obtain enough information to understand the basic actions on the body for these medications.

Digitalis medications like digoxin are indicated for congestive heart failure (CHF). They work by increasing the force of the heart contraction. Digoxin levels may need to be monitored. If the digoxin level is too high, it could cause lowered heart rate among other things. If this overload does occur, the drug Digibind or an equivalent can be given. This causes the excess digoxin to bind to the antidote and be passed off as waste.

* Lanoxin – Digoxin

Anti-arrhythmic agents are used to treat abnormalities in the cardiac rhythm. Arrhythmias can be detected by an electrocardiogram (EKG). They can lessen the heart's ability to pump blood efficiently or even at all. Basically, the goal for all these agents is to get the heart beating in a rhythm as close to normal as possible and maintain it there.

* Xylocaine - Lidocaine
* Cordarone – Amiodarone
* Mexitil – Mexiletine

Calcium channel blockers work differently than other angina agents. They inhibit the movement of calcium into both heart muscle and smooth vascular muscles. Without the calcium, coronary arteries are dilated, which in turn decreases the force of the contraction and the demand for oxygen.

* Procardia - Nifedipine
* Norvasc – Amlodipine
* Cardizem – Diltiazem
* Calan – Verapamil

Vasodilators are indicated for acute angina or angina prophylaxis. These medications do exactly as their drug class says: They dilate the "vaso" or the blood vessels. When there is an increased area through which the blood can travel, naturally there will be less pressure built up behind it. Nitroglycerin is one of the most potent and commonly used vasodilators. For an acute angina attack, nitroglycerin can be used to dilate the vessels rapidly. In addition to vasodilatation, these meds cause retention of salt and water. Using a diuretic medication offsets this side affect.

* Isordil   – Isosorbide Dinitrate
* Nitrostat   – Nitroglycerin Sublingual
* Apresoline – Hydralazine

Beta-blockers are indicated for hypertension, angina pectoris and migraine prophylaxis among others. They compete with beta agonists for receptor sites. These drugs inhibit the vasodilator response to beta-adrenergic stimulation.

* Tenormin – Atenolol
* Lopressor – Metoprolol
* Inderal – Propranolol

The Angiotensin Converting Enzyme (ACE) needed to produce Angiotensin II causes severe vasoconstriction. The class of medications called **ACE inhibitors** inhibits the Angiotensin Converting Enzyme; therefore less Angiotensin II is produced causing less vasoconstriction and lower blood pressure.

* Capoten – Captopril
* Vasotec – Enalapril
* Prinivil – Lisinopril

Diuretics are given for edema and/or hypertension in combination with other antihypertensives. Thiazide diuretics increase urinary excretion of sodium and chloride. They also inhibit the reabsorption of these in the kidneys. Loop diuretics also inhibit the reabsorption of sodium and chloride.

* Lozol – Indapamide
* Hygroton – Chlorthalidone
* Lasix – Furosemide
* Demedex – Torsemide
* Zaroxolyn – Metolazone

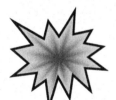

Math Blaster

For the Mission 10 Math Blaster, feel free to review the explanations in Mission 5 for the pharmacy calculations. In the mission 10 debriefing, you will be revisiting the skills learned in the earlier Mission.

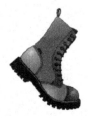

Drill Practice

For this mission's drill practice, rework those questions found in Mission 5 drill practice. In the Mission 10 debriefing, you will be checking to see how well you remember those skills.

Drug Training Chapter Eleven

Brand Name	Generic Name	Drug Classification	Primary Indication	Side effects, Warnings, Other
Aricept	Donepezil	Acetylcholinesterase inhibitor	Dementia, Alzheimer's	nausea, diarrhea, insomnia, vomiting, muscle cramp, fatigue and anorexia.
Niaspan	Niacin	Antihyperlipidemic	Hypercholesterolemia	flushing, diarrhea, nausea, vomiting, increased cough and pruritus
Byetta	Exenatide Injection	Incretin Mimetic	Type 2 Diabetes	Note: Byetta is not an insulin - substitute. May cause GI upset primarily nausea, dizziness, jitters
Fosamax	Alendronate	Bisphosphonate	Osteoporosis treatment and prevention	Must be taken upon rising for the day and at least 30 minutes before eating or drinking with plain water only then patients should not lie down for at least 30 minutes and until after their first food of the day. Most side effects are gastric related.
Combivent	Ipratropium/ albuterol	Bronchdilator	Chronic Obstructive Pulmonary Disease (COPD)	Headache, Bronchitis and other upper respiratory disturbances including cough
Diabeta	glyburide	sulfonylurea glucose lowering agent	type 2 diabetes mellitus	hypoglycemia, nausea, epigastric fullness, and heartburn
Prevacid	Lansoprazole	Proton-Pump Inhibitor	Gastric ulcer, Esophagitis, Gastroesophageal Reflux Disease (GERD)	Abdominal pain, nausea, vomiting, diarrhea, constipation, headache
Lopid	Gemfibrozil	Lipid regulating Agent	Hypertriglyceridemia	Dyspepsia, abdominal pain, nausea and vomiting, diarrhea, headache

Brand Name	Generic Name	Drug Classification	Primary Indication	Side effects, Warnings, Other
Lantus	Glargine insulin	recombinant human insulin analog.	Types I and II Diabetes Mellitus	Hypoglycemia, Hypokalemia, pain, itching or redness at the injection site.
Xalatan	Lantanoprost	Glaucoma agent	Intraocular pressure with glaucoma or ocular hypertension	Eyelash changes, eyelid skin darkening; intraocular inflammation, iris pigmentation changes, macular edema, must be refrigerated
Adderall	Amphetamine/ Dextroamphetamine mixed salts	C II CNS Stimulant	Attention Deficit Hyperactivity Disorder (ADHD) and Narcolepsy.	Palpitations, tachycardia, hypertension, overstimulation, restlessness, dizziness, insomnia, euphoria, loss of appetite
Naprosyn	Naproxen	Non-Steroidal Anti-Inflammatory Drug (NSAID)	Mild to moderate pain, dysmenorrhea, osteoarthritis, rheumatoid arthritis, spondylitis and other joint related disorders	May increase risk of serious cardiovascular thrombotic events, myocardial infarction, stroke and GI bleeding; may also cause

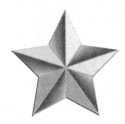

Mission 11 Debriefing

Answer the following questions in assessment of the lessons learned in Mission 11. For best results, repeat the exercise until no questions are missed then move on to the next mission.

1. Nitroglycerin is a very powerful and commonly used _____.
    a) anti-arrhythmic agent
    b) vasodilator
    c) calcium channel blocker
    d) digitalis agent

2. The digestive system is how nutrients and oxygen are carried to individual cell tissues as well as how wastes and carbon dioxide are removed from those cell tissues.
    a) True
    b) False

3. The drug Adderall is a _____ controlled substance.
    a) C V
    b) C IV
    c) C III
    d) C II

4. An overload of digitalis medication can _____ a patient's heart rate.
    a) Increase
    b) Decrease
    c) Will not affect
    d) None of these

5. The contraction phase of the heart is referred to as the _____ and gives top number of the blood pressure reading.
    a) diastole
    b) systole
    c) bystole
    d) triastole

6. An order for 1 pound of 5% zinc oxide paste is prepared using the pharmacy's stock 10% paste and 2% paste. How much of the 2% stock paste must be mixed to obtain the desired concentration?
    a) 180g
    b) 300g
    c) 480g
    d) 280g

7. About _____ of blood is plasma which is mostly water.
    a) 35%
    b) 45%
    c) 55%
    d) 65%

8. Arterial walls are thicker and much more rigid than venular walls.
    a) True
    b) False

9. Angiotensin II causes _____.
   a) Vasoconstriction
   b) Increased blood pressure
   c) Both a and b
   d) Neither a nor b

10. Which of the following agents is a cholinesterase inhibitor?
   a) Fosamax
   b) Aricept
   c) Lantus
   d) Lopid

11. A white blood cell is also known as a(n)_____.
   a) Platelet
   b) Erythrocyte
   c) Emcyte
   d) Leukocyte

12. To process a prescription order for a 7.5% dextrose solution, the pharmacy technician would mix the on hand stock of 10% dextrose and water to make one Liter of the 7.5% solution? How much of the 10% stock solution will be needed?
   a) 750mL
   b) 500mL
   c) 250mL
   d) 400mL

13. The _____ is the largest artery.
   a) Superior vena cava
   b) Aorta
   c) Pulmonary artery
   d) None of these

14. Cordarone and Mexitil are both _____.
   a) Beta Blockers
   b) Alpha Blockers
   c) Calcium Channel Blockers
   d) None of these

15. Which of the following can be found in blood plasma?
   a) Proteins
   b) Antibodies
   c) Hormones
   d) Nutrients
   e) Only a and c
   f) All of these

16. There are normally about _____ of blood flowing through the cardiovascular system at any given time.
   a) 14 pints
   b) 11 pints
   c) 4 pints
   d) 8 pints

17. Byetta is an insulin substitute.
   a) True
   b) False

18. _____ are given to treat edema or swelling.
   a) Vasodilators
   b) Diuretics
   c) Calcium channel blockers
   d) ACE inhibitors

19. Both Capoten and Vasotec are ACE inhibiting drugs.
   a) True
   b) False

20. The drug Prinivil is classified as a(n) _____.
 a) diuretic
 c) ACE inhibitor
 b) vasodilator
 d) beta-blocker

21. Regulation of vasoconstriction and vasodilation is controlled by the _____.
 a) Central nervous system
 b) Autonomic nervous system

22. The povidone iodine solution your pharmacy stocks is 10%. A patient brings a script for 3% povidone iodine solution, 8 oz to use as directed. How much 10% stock solution will you need to compound this mixture?
 a) 120mL
 c) 40mL
 b) 168mL
 d) 72mL

23. The drug furosemide is classified as an ACE inhibitor.
 a) True
 b) False

24. The heart muscle is directly supplied fresh oxygen by the network of _____ arteries.
 a) cardial
 c) coronary
 b) coronary sinus
 d) pulmonary

25. All but which of the following drugs are indicated for patients who have diabetes?
 a) Glyburide
 c) Exenatide injection
 b) Lantanoprost
 d) Glargine insulin

26. Vasodilators cause fluid retention and often require the use of a diuretic.
 a) True
 b) False

27. Red blood cells typically outnumber white blood cells approximately _____ to 1.
 a) 300
 c) 700
 b) 500
 d) 1000

28. Red blood cells can also be called erythrocytes.
 a) True
 b) False

29. Digitalis medications are indicated for patients who have _____
 a) high blood pressure
 c) high cholesterol levels
 b) diabetes
 d) congestive heart failure

30. _____ assist in blood clotting which is also called coagulation.
 a) Platelets
 c) Red blood cells
 b) White blood cells
 d) None of these

31. The pharmacy has a 20% strength and a 5% strength of the same ointment. An order comes in for 4oz of 12% ointment. How much 5% ointment would be needed?
 a) 56g
 c) 64g
 b) 80g
 d) 40g

32. The heart pumps about _____ through itself in a single day's time.
    a) 2,000-3,000
    b) 5,000-6.000
    c) 10,000 – 12,000
    d) 80,000 – 90,000

33. There are four kinds of blood cells.
    a) True
    b) False

34. In the _____ is where the oxygen exchange for the tissues takes place.
    a) Arteries
    b) Heart
    c) Veins
    d) Capillaries

35. Lantanoprost should be stored _____.
    a) in the freezer
    b) under refrigeration
    c) at room temperature
    d) in a warm place

36. Which of the following is not a calcium channel blocker?
    a) Amlodipine
    b) Diltiazem
    c) Verapamil
    d) None of these

37. Antiarrythmic agents treat abnormalities in cardiac rhythm, or irregular heartbeats.
    a) True
    b) False

38. What should the final product be labeled if 200mL of metronidazole suspension contains 4.8 grams of active ingredient?
    a) 0.024%
    b) 41.6%
    c) 2.4%
    d) 9.6%

39. Though calcium channel blockers, vasodilators and beta-blockers are from different classifications, they can all be used to treat _____.
    a) arrhythmias
    b) angina
    c) high cholesterol
    d) fluid overload

40. The blood pressure is stronger in the arteries than it is in the _____.
    a) Veins
    b) Capillaries
    c) Both a and b
    d) Neither a nor b

41. The drug Prevacid is an H_2 antagonist drug.
    a) True
    b) False

42. Which of the following pairs of drugs are both beta-blockers?
    a) Tenormin and Inderal
    b) Isordil and Apresoline
    c) Norvasc and Calan
    d) Lopressor and Cardizem

43. The stock oral suspension contains 5 grams of active ingredient in 125ml of suspension? What should be labeled as the strength of this mixture?
    a) 0.04%
    b) 40%
    c) 5%
    d) 4%

44. The _____ is the only artery to carry low oxygen blood.
    a) coronary artery
    b) pulmonary artery
    c) aorta
    d) vena cava

45. If blood types are not cross-matched properly from donor to receiver it can be detrimental to the receiving patient by causing the blood to clump up.
    a) True
    b) False

46. The lungs replenish carbon dioxide and remove and expell oxygen from the blood.
    a) True
    b) False

47. A patient just dropped off a prescription that could not be written with refills. Which of the following must have been written for that patient?
    a) Naprosyn
    b) Adderall
    c) Lantus
    d) Fosamax

48. Which of the following blood cells helps to protect the body from harmful organisms?
    a) Leukocytes
    b) Erythrocytes
    c) Platelets
    d) Red blood cells

49. Many larger, longer veins have one-way valves inside to prevent the backflow of blood.
    a) True
    b) False

50. You have 20ml of a 1:200 solution in stock. If the pharmacist has asked you to dilute the solution to 480ml, how would you label the final strength?
    a) 0.02%
    b) 0.12%
    c) 12%
    d) 24%

51. The aorta is approximately one-fourth of an inch in diameter.
    a) True
    b) False

52. Alendronate is classified as a(n) _____.
    a) proton pump inhibitor
    b) cholinesterase inhibitor
    c) bisphosphonate
    d) bronchodilator

53. Zaroxolyn and Lozol are both classified as _____.
    a) ACE inhibitors
    b) ARB blockers
    c) diuretics
    d) calcium channel blockers

54. If 300ml of a 15% solution are diluted to 1000ml, what will the final percent strength be?
    a) 0.045%
    b) 4.5%
    c) 0.5%
    d) 5%

55. The blood passes through the _____ valve as it moves from the left atrium to the left ventricle.
    a) Mitral
    b) Pulmonary
    c) Tricuspid
    d) None of these

56. What volume of 5% solution will be needed to make 120ml of a 0.6% solution?
    a) 1.4mL
    b) 100mL
    c) 10mL
    d) 14.4mL

57. Blood pressure is measured by a device called a _____.
    a) Thermometer
    b) Glucometer
    c) Sphygmomanometer
    d) None of these

58. You have 40ml of a 1:10 solution in stock. If the pharmacist has asked you to dilute the solution to 3%, how many milliliters can be prepared?
    a) 120mL
    b) 133mL
    c) 1200mL
    d) 142mL

59. Naproxen may increase the risk of serious cardiovascular events including myocardial infarction, stroke and also GI bleeding.
    a) True
    b) False

60. There are about _____ miles of blood vessels in the body.
    a) 5,000
    b) 6,000
    c) 50,000
    d) 90,000

61. Many cells will pass through the _____ in single file because of the small diameter of the vessels.
    a) Veins
    b) Capillaries
    c) Arteries
    d) Lungs

62. Which of the following is true concerning the use of Fosamax?
    a) After taking, patients should not lie down for at least 30 minutes.
    b) The medication should be taken when the patient first wakes up for the day.
    c) Eating or drinking should not be done for at least 30 minutes (other than taking with water)
    d) All of these statements are true.

63. The heart muscle is sometimes called the _____.
    a) Pulmonarium
    b) Myocardium
    c) Lymphatocardiac muscle
    d) None of these

64. Naproxen is classified as a CNS stimulant.
    a) True
    b) False

65. Which of the following dumps directly into the right atrium?
    a) Coronary artery
    b) Vena cava
    c) Both a and b
    d) Neither a nor b

66. If 6oz of ibuprofen ointment contains 20g of ibuprofen, with what strength should the package be labeled?
    a) 9%
    b) 3%
    c) 11%
    d) 30%

67. There are only _____ different blood types.
   a) Two
   c) Six
   b) Four
   d) Three

68. Which pairs of drugs below are indicated to treat patients with some form of high cholesterol?
   a) Niaspan and Fosamax
   c) Diabeta and Fosamax
   b) Diabeta and Lopid
   d) Niaspan and Lopid

69. The brief moment of relaxation in between heartbeats is called a diastole and gives the reading for the bottom number in a blood pressure.
   a) True
   b) False

70. If the technician has prepared a 480g jar of sugardine ointment for use in the wound care center, how many grams of 10% povidone iodine ointment were included if the final strength is labeled at 4%?
   a) 192g
   c) 19.2g
   b) 120g
   d) 12g

71. The _____ brings blood from the body back to the heart.
   a) Aorta
   c) Vena cava
   b) Pulmonary artery
   d) Pulmonary vein

72. An asthma patient has just visited the clinic and was prescribed a bronchodilator. Which of the following may have been prescribed for the patient?
   a) Aricept
   c) Combivent
   b) Adderall
   d) Diabeta

73. Digibind can be given if a patient's blood level of digoxin gets too high.
   a) True
   b) False

74. The blood passes through the _____ valve as it moves from the right atrium to the right ventricle.
   a) Mitral
   c) Bicuspid
   b) Pulmonary
   d) Tricuspid

75. Hydralazine is known as a(n) _____.
   a) ACE inhibitor
   c) digitalis agent
   b) vasodilator
   d) calcium channel blocker

76. The cardiovascular system is the major transportation system within the body tissues.
   a) True
   b) False

Match the following drugs to their generic names.

77. Naprosyn   _____ a) donepezil
78. Xalatan   _____ b) niacin
79. Lopid   _____ c) exenatide injection
80. Diabeta   _____ d) alendronate
81. Fosamax   _____ e) ipratropium/albuterol
82. Niaspan   _____ f) gemfibrozil
83. Aricept   _____ g) glyburide
84. Byetta   _____ h) lansoprazole
85. Combivent   _____ i) naproxen
86. Adderall   _____ j) glargine insulin
87. Lantus   _____ k) lantanoprost
88. Prevacid   _____ l) amphetamine/dextroamphetamine mixed salts

Match the following drugs to their classifications.

89. Exenatide injection   _____ a) Cholinesterase inhibitor
90. Ipratropium/albuterol   _____ b) lipid regulating agent
91. Lansoprazole   _____ c) incretin mimetic
92. Glyburide   _____ d) recombinant human insulin analog
93. Alendronate   _____ e) CNS stimulant
94. Niacin   _____ f) NSAID
95. Gemfibrozil   _____ g) glaucoma agent
96. Donepezil   _____ h) sulfonylurea
97. Glargine insulin   _____ i) bronchodilator
98. Lantanoprost   _____ j) bisphosphonate
99. Naproxen   _____ k) proton pump inhibitor
100. Amphetamine/   _____ l) antihyperlipidemic
Dextroamphetamine
Mixed salts

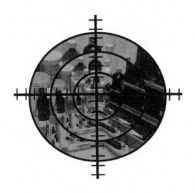

Mission 12
The Respiratory System
Medications and Malfunctions

Mission Objectives

*To understand the basic anatomy and physiology of the respiratory system and its components.

*To learn of the drug families used in treating respiratory disorders.

*To understand the pharmacology of drugs used in treating respiratory disorders.

*To gain baseline knowledge of twelve of the most popular drugs on the market.

*To review pharmacy business calculations.

The **respiratory system** is in control of bringing in fresh oxygen to the blood and expelling carbon dioxide. The air around us holds the oxygen the body needs and the **lungs** are the breathing machines the body uses to take it in. The respiratory system is composed of the nose, pharynx, larynx, trachea, bronchi, bronchioles, alveoli and the lungs. The **lungs** are the sponge-like structures that enclose the entire bronchial tree. The lungs are divided into **lobes**. The right lung has three lobes and is larger than the left lung. The left lung has only two lobes. Since it is smaller it leaves room for the heart. The respiratory system is divided into two parts: upper and lower.

External respiration is the airflow in and out of the lungs. As the air is inhaled, it must first travel through the **upper respiratory tract**. This consists of the **nose, pharynx** and **larynx**. Here in the upper respiratory tract air is filtered, moistened and warmed. The inhaled air continues through the upper respiratory tract and enters the **lower respiratory tract** that begins at the trachea.

The **trachea** branches into two major **bronchi**, one for each lung. Air will follow one path or the other and enter even smaller bronchi then **bronchioles**. These bronchioles end in **alveoli** or air sacs. The alveoli are actually what make up most of the lung tissue. They are what fill with air and expand as the body inhales. Approximately 150 million of these alveoli are in each average adult lung.

As air enters these alveoli, it comes in very close contact with the capillaries filled with blood. The thin walls of the capillaries allow for the exchange of gases. Oxygen molecules are absorbed by the fluid in the alveolus lining. The **oxygen** passes to the blood through the thin alveolus wall and attaches to the hemoglobin molecules of red blood cells. Meanwhile, **carbon dioxide** is passed from the blood though the thin walls of the alveolus where it can be exhaled from the body. This entire gas exchange process is known as **internal respiration**.

The carbon dioxide level in the blood determines the breathing rate. The more carbon dioxide that is in the blood, the more acidic the blood will be. During rest periods when the carbon dioxide level is low, the breathing rate slows way down. During periods of activity the acid level rises and the breathing reflex is stimulated to breathe deeper and more rapidly. This is monitored and controlled by the respiratory centers in the brain, particularly the one located in the medulla oblongata.

The lungs and inner walls of the thoracic cavity are completely surrounded by an airtight sac called the **pleura**. This pleura secretes fluid that lubricates and helps to keep the pleural layers from causing friction against the chest wall.

As inspiration takes place, the muscles of the **diaphragm** contract pulling it downward, expanding the chest cavity. At the same time, the intercostal muscles of the ribcage contract pulling the ribs outward and upward. This makes a vacuum and forces air into the lungs. As expiration occurs, it reverses the act of the inspiration. The diaphragm relaxes and rises. Also the muscles around the ribs relax forcing them downward and inward. This pushes air in the lungs to be expelled from the body.

The body depends on normal respiratory function to provide the blood with fresh oxygen. If it is impaired in any way, breathing is difficult and the body might suffer from too little oxygen, which can cause severe health problems. There are many different types of lung disorders or illnesses.

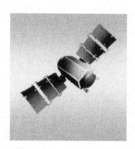

Recon Mission 12:

There are so many different diseases that can be associated with the respiratory system. With this mission's reconnaissance you are encouraged to search the Internet for information on various diseases and disorders of the respiratory system. Also seek out anatomical diagrams of the respiratory system so that each area becomes more familiar to you now that a review of the functionality has been completed. Many websites offer interactive diagrams which allow you to label and maneuver them.

Write down as many of the conditions as you can find with a brief description of each one. As you continue on this mission, some medications may be discussed that are used primarily to treat diseases and disorders that you have read about and familiarized yourself with. As a guide only, the following bulleted points could be used as keywords in your search. Each keyword suggested below may have multiple possible inclusions for your review. You are encouraged to devote plenty of time to this activity.

* Respiratory System diseases and disorders
* Respiratory illnesses
* Interactive diagrams of the Respiratory System

Medications for Malfunctions

There are many drug classes that affect the respiratory system. Here you will learn of the basic classes and their pharmacological actions on the body. Take into consideration that true pharmacology goes much deeper than you will learn in this preparatory course, but you should obtain enough information to understand the basic actions on the body for these medications.

Bronchodilators do exactly what their name says. They dilate the bronchioles. They relax the smooth muscles of the bronchial walls to reverse bronchospasm caused by asthma, exercise-induced bronchospasm, bronchitis, emphysema or other pulmonary illnesses.

* Ventolin – Albuterol
* Proventil – Albuterol
* Alupent – Metaproterenol Sulfate
* Theo-Dur – Theophylline
* Atrovent – Ipratropium Bromide

Leukotriene receptor antagonists are indicated for treatment of chronic asthma and the prophylaxis of it. These medicines inhibit bronchoconstriction.

* Accolate – Zafirlukast
* Singulair – Montelukast

Some respiratory inhalants are **corticosteroids**. These inhalants are adrenocortical steroids with basic glucocorticoid actions. This type of inhaler most likely decreases the number and activity of anti-inflammatory cells, inhibits bronchoconstriction, and relaxes smooth muscle among other things. The inhaler can provide local corticosteroid effects without many other systemic effects.

* Pulmicort – Budesonide
* Aerobid – Flunisolide
* Azmacort – Triamcinolone
* Beclovent – Beclomethasone
* Vanceril – Beclomethasone
* Flovent – Fluticasone

There are nasal inhalers that have basically the same effects on the nasal membranes, as do the oral inhalers on the mucous membranes in the lungs. Most of them have the same active ingredient in a different dosage form.

Nasal decongestants offer relief of temporary nasal congestion due to colds, hay fever and/or upper respiratory allergies. These medications cause vasoconstriction of mucus membranes. The shrinkage of these membranes causes drainage, which improves ventilation and relieves the stuffiness. Patients with severe hypertension should use this type of medication only under a doctor's supervision due to the vasoconstriction and possibility of increased blood pressure.

* Sudafed – Pseudoephedrine
* Neo-Synephrine – Phenylephrine
* Afrin – Oxymetazoline

The Combat Meth Act now requires that all products that contain the ingredient of pseudoephedrine be placed behind the pharmacy counter. Currently, in most states, these products are still available without a prescription but a logbook, either manual or electronic, must be kept with a record of sales, to whom, how much and how often. Some states are now considering pseudoephedrine containing products as a controlled substance and in those states a prescription would be required. Patients must always follow the laws within their state.

Antihistamines are widely used for an array of effects. They have varying degrees of antihistaminic, anticholinergic, sedative, antiemetic, antitussive effects and several other uses. Antihistamines are competitive reversible H_1 receptor antagonists. They reduce or prevent the majority of the physiologic effects that histamine normally induces at the H_1 receptor site. Although they do not affect the release of histamine; they will block its action at the receptor site. This action will ultimately reduce the wheal, flare and itch response most likely to be associated with allergic or histaminic reactions.

Though both codeine and dextromethorphan are available as a sole ingredient, both are included in many other anti-tussives.
Those products containing often include AC or DM respectively, as part of the drug name.

Also an anti-inflammatory response in nasal mucous will induce a release of histamines that are powerful vasodilators. This vasodilation causes excessive mucous secretion, sneezing and congestion. Therefore, antihistamines would be most effective in treatment of allergic rhinitis. Antihistamines consequently reduce the amount of mucous secretions and cause a drying effect.

* Chlor-Trimeton – Chlorpheniramine
* Benadryl – Diphenhydramine
* Atarax – Hydroxyzine HCl
* Zyrtec – Cetirizine
* Claritin – Loratadine
* Allegra – Fexofenadine

Antitussives are given to treat non-productive cough when there is no presence of mucous in the respiratory tract. The cough suppressant action is gained from a direct action on the cough center in the medulla oblongata.

* Tessalon Perles - Benzonatate
* Delsym - Dextromethorphan

Expectorants are given to relieve respiratory conditions with a non-productive cough and the presence of mucous in the respiratory tract. Expectorants work by enhancing the output of fluid in the respiratory tract, thus helping to liquefy the mucous and ease its expulsion. Expectorants help to turn a non-productive cough into a productive one.

* Robitussin – Guaifenesin
* Mucinex - Guaifenesin

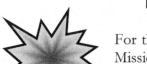

Math Blaster

For the Mission 12 Math Blaster, feel free to review the explanations in Mission 7 for the pharmacy calculations. In the mission 12 debriefing, you will be revisiting the skills learned in the earlier Mission.

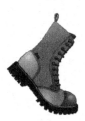

Drill Practice

For this mission's drill practice, rework those questions found in Mission 7 drill practice. In the Mission 12 debriefing, you will be checking to see how well you remember those skills.

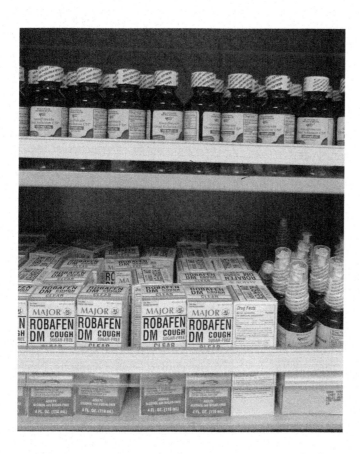

Drug Training Chapter Twelve

Brand Name	Generic Name	Drug Classification	Primary Indication	Side effects, Warnings, Other
Indocin	Indomethacin	NSAID	rheumatoid arthritis, spondylitis, osteoarthritis, gouty arthritis, bursitis, tendinitis	increased risk of serious cardiovascular thrombotic events, myocardial infarction, stroke and GI bleeding nausea, vomiting, dyspepsia, headache, dizziness,
Valtrex	valacyclovir	Antiviral	Genital herpes, cold sores, chickenpox, shingles	headache, nausea, and abdominal pain
Mobic	Meloxicam	NSAID	osteoarthritis, rheumatoid arthritis	increased risk of serious cardiovascular thrombotic events, myocardial infarction, stroke, GI bleeding, ulceration, and perforation of the stomach or intestines which can be fatal
Vyvanse	lisdexamfetamine	CII CNS Stimulant	Attention Deficit Hyperactivity Disorder	ventricular hypertrophy, tic, vomiting, psychomotor hyperactivity, insomnia, rash, irritability, decreased appetite
Abilify	aripiprazole	Antipsychotic	schizophrenia, bipolar I disorder, major depressive disorder,	increased risk of death in elderly patients with dementia-related psychosis treated with antipsychotic drugs
Omnicef	cefdinir	extended-spectrum, semisynthetic cephalosporin	mild to moderate infections caused by susceptible strains	Diarrhea, vaginal moniliasis, Headache, Nausea, abdominal pain
Lyrica	pregabalin	anticonvulsant though primarily used as neuropathic agent	neuralgia	dizziness, somnolence, dizziness, blurry vision, weight gain, sleepiness, trouble concentrating, swelling of your hands and feet, dry mouth, and feeling "high

Brand Name	Generic Name	Drug Classification	Primary Indication	Side effects, Warnings, Other
Lanoxin	digoxin	cardiac glycoside/ digitalis agent	congestive heart failure, ventricular response rate with chronic atrial fibrillation	heart block , anorexia, nausea, vomiting, diarrhea, headache, weakness, dizziness, apathy, confusion, blurred vision and mental disturbances
Atarax, Vistaril	Hydroxyzine	antihistamine, anti-anxiety agent,	pruritus, chronic urticaria, anxiety	Drowsiness, dry mouth
Coreg	Carvedilol	Beta-adrenergic blocker	mild-to-severe chronic heart failure	dizziness,fatigue, asthenia, bradycardia, hypotension, diarrhrea, nausea and vomiting, cough, hyperglycemia
Detrol LA	Tolterodine	antimuscarinic	overactive bladder , urinary incontinence, urgency, and frequency	dry mouth, headache, constipation, abdominal pain, abnormal vision,urinary retention, and dry eyes
Keflex	Cephalexin	Cephalosporin antibiotic	treats infection of susceptible strains including both Streptococcus and Staphylococcus among others	diarrhea, dyspepsia, gastritis, abdominal pain, pruritus, rash

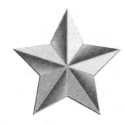

Mission 12 Debriefing

Answer the following questions in assessment of the lessons learned in Mission 12. For best results, repeat the exercise until no questions are missed then move on to the next mission.

1. Which of the following drugs puts patients at increased risk of serious cardiovascular events such as stroke, heart attack, blood clots and GI bleeding?
   a) Lisdexamfetamine
   b) Indomethacin
   c) Pregabalin
   d) Aripiprazole

2. A bag of adult diapers costs the pharmacy $14.50 and earns a profit of 35%. What is the retail price of the diapers?
   a) $17.19
   b) $5.08
   c) $21.27
   d) $19.58

3. The right lung with 3 lobes is larger than the left lung with only 2 lobes.
   a) True
   b) False

4. The drug Vyvanse is a _____ controlled substance.
   a) C II
   b) C III
   c) C IV
   d) C V

5. A batch of prescriptions totals $46.18 and a patient pays with a hundred dollar bill. How many of which denominations should be given in change?
   a) 2 twenties, 1 five, 3 ones, 3 quarters, 1 dime and 2 pennies.
   b) 2 twenties, 1 ten, 3 ones, 3 quarters, 1 dime and 2 pennies.
   c) 2 twenties, 1 ten, 4 ones, 3 quarters, 1 dime and 3 pennies.
   d) 2 twenties, 1 ten, 1 five, 3 ones, 3 quarters, 1 dime and 2 pennies.

6. Both Omnicef and Keflex are grouped into which class of antibacterials for infection?
   a) Penicillins
   b) Cephalosporins
   c) Fluoroquinolones
   d) Macrolides

7. A beauty product currently earns the pharmacy a hefty 38% profit margin. If the item costs $20.00 how much does it retail for?
   a) $7.60
   b) $12.40
   c) $29.70
   d) $27.60

8. Which of the following medications is an antihistamine and will cause drowsiness.
   a) Dextromethorphan
   b) Diphenhydramine
   c) Guaifenesin
   d) None of these

9. The respiratory system is responsible for bringing fresh carbon dioxide to the blood and removing oxygen from the blood as it passes through the lungs.
   a) True
   b) False

10. Though _____ is an anticonvulsant, it is primarily indicated to treat neuropathy.
    a) Mobic
    b) Valtrex
    c) Vyvanse
    d) Lyrica

11. A customer owes $60.37 for all purchases and hands the cashier four twenties. What is the value of the change?
    a) $19.63
    b) $39.63
    c) $9.63
    d) $29.63

12. The airflow in and out of the lungs is known as _____.
    a) alveolar respiration
    b) internal respiration
    c) external respiration
    d) none of these

13. A daily pill box is on sale this week only for 15% off its regular retail price of $12.29. What would the customer have to pay for this item?
    a) $1.84
    b) $14.13
    c) $10.92
    d) $10.45

14. The trachea is included in the lower respiratory tract.
    a) True
    b) False

15. A patient with hypertension and chronic heart failure has been prescribed a beta-blocker. Which of the medications listed is found in this class and could have been prescribed?
    a) Lanoxin
    b) Lyrica
    c) Coreg
    d) Atarax

16. A discontinued digital blood pressure cuff is being marked down 40%. If it used to retail for $78.99, what is its new price?
    a) $31.60
    b) $47.39
    c) $43.44
    d) $35.55

17. Which of the following organs is included in the upper respiratory tract?
    a) Trachea
    b) Bronchi
    c) Pharynx
    d) Bronchioles

18. A generic store brand pain reliever earns 25% for the pharmacy. Its cost is $2.30 so what would the selling price need to be set at?
    a) $2.88
    b) $0.58
    c) $1.73
    d) $3.19

19. Elderly patients with dementia related psychosis who are prescribed the drug, Abilify, are at an increased risk of _____.
   a) GI bleeding
   b) blood clots and strokes
   c) suicidal thoughts
   d) death

20. In the lower respiratory tract, air is filtered, moistened and warmed.
   a) True
   b) False

21. A shower chair is on clearance and has a markdown of 90%. The regular retail price was $72.49. How much would the sale price be?
   a) $65.29
   b) $7.92
   c) $7.25
   d) $5.80

22. Aripiprazole is classified as a(n) _____.
   a) Antipsychotic
   b) Antihistamine
   c) Proton Pump inhibitor
   d) ACE inhibitor

23. A low priced item earns a profit of 54% for the pharmacy. If the acquisition cost sits at $2.80, what is the actual retail price of the item?
   a) $1.51
   b) $4.31
   c) $1.29
   d) $6.20

24. The diaphragm relaxes and rises as _____ occurs.
   a) Inspiration
   b) Expiration
   c) Coughing
   d) None of these

25. A new bottle of vitamins costs just $7.80. The pharmacy needs to gain 30% profit on the item. What is the markup value?
   a) $2.34
   b) $10.14
   c) $5.46
   d) $3.82

26. Some states are now requiring a prescription to obtain pseudoephedrine products.
   a) True
   b) False

27. A patient's bill for meds rings up at $32.13 but all the patient has is a hundred dollar bill. How many of which denominations should be given in change?
   a) 3 twenties, 1 ten, 2 ones, 3 quarters, 1 dime, and 2 pennies
   b) 3 twenties, 1 five, 2 ones, 3 quarters, 1 dime, and 2 pennies
   c) 2 twenties, 1 five, 2 ones, 3 quarters, 1 dime, and 2 pennies
   d) 3 twenties, 1 five, 4 ones, 3 quarters, 1 dime, and 2 pennies

28. There are about _____ alveoli in each adult lung.
   a) 150 million
   b) 5 to 6 thousand
   c) 5 to 6 million
   d) 300 million

29. Antitussives act directly on the cough center in the _____.
   a) Throat
   c) Medulla
   b) Lungs
   d) Gut

30. Which of the following drugs is a leukotriene receptor antagonist?
   a) Sudafed
   c) Azmacort
   b) Singulair
   d) Atrovent

31. A shower chair has an acquisition cost of $78.00 but earns a 20% profit for the pharmacy. What is the current retail price of this item?
   a) $15.60
   c) $93.60
   b) $108.60
   d) $23.60

32. Which of the following medications is indicated for patients with overactive bladder issues?
   a) Valcyclovir
   c) Tolteradine
   b) Aripiprazole
   d) Cephalexin

33. The diaphragm _____ during inhalation or inspiration.
   a) relaxes and rises
   c) is not affected
   b) contracts pulling downward
   d) is stretched to its peak

34. A item is on sale this week only for 15% off its regular retail price of $14.99 What would the customer have to pay for this item?
   a) $2.25
   c) $11.18
   b) $10.76
   d) $12.74

35. The amount of oxygen in the blood determines the breathing rate.
   a) True
   b) False

36. The airtight sac surrounding the lungs is known as the _____.
   a) pulmocardium
   c) pleura
   b) pnuemocardium
   d) pulmonary sac

37. A sale for $2.22 is paid for with a five dollar bill. What should be given in returned change?
   a) 2 ones, 3 quarters, 3 pennies
   c) 2 ones, 2 dimes, 2 pennies
   b) 3 ones, 3 quarters, 3 pennies
   d) 2 ones, 3 dimes, 3 pennies

38. An inhaled corticosteroid can offer the benefits of steroid use without the common systemic effects since those effects would remain local to the mucous membranes.
   a) True
   b) False

39. A thermometer costs $7.00 and gains a 30% profit. What is its retail price?
   a) $10.00
   c) $9.10
   b) $2.10
   d) $4.90

40. The drug digoxin is primarily indicated for patients who have which of these conditions?
    a) Depression
    b) Congestive heart failure
    c) Hypertension
    d) Schizophrenia

41. _____ are given to relieve cough when it is non-productive and there is no mucous.
    a) Expectorants
    b) Antitussives
    c) Leukotriene receptor antagonists
    d) Antihistamines

42. A weight loss supplement currently sells for $22.49 per bottle. The pharmacy pays only $15.00 cost on the product. What is the profit margin earned when someone purchases this item?
    a) 33.3%
    b) 66.7%
    c) 49.9%
    d) 42.6%

43. Which of the following is not included in the lower respiratory tract?
    a) Larynx
    b) Trachea
    c) Bronchioles
    d) Bronchi

44. An item currently retailing for $39.99 is on sale at 30% off. What is the new sale price of the item?
    a) $27.99
    b) $11.99
    c) $12.00
    d) $51.99

45. Guaifenesin is a commonly used antitussive.
    a) True
    b) False

46. An item earns a whopping 65% profit but only costs a mere $8.00. What would the selling price need to be to ensure this profit percentage?
    a) $5.20
    b) $13.20
    c) $12.78
    d) $14.82

47. Which of the following is a decongestant and could offer relief of nasal congestion?
    a) Phenylephrine
    b) Guaifenesin
    c) Diphenhydramine
    d) None of these

48. An item retailing for $50.39 is being marked down 25%. What is the new discounted price of the item?
    a) $37.79
    b) $12.60
    c) $35.27
    d) $15.12

49. _____ can increase blood pressure so patients with severe hypertension should only use this class of medications under a physician's care.
    a) Antihistamines
    b) Expectorants
    c) Antitussives
    d) Nasal decongestants

50. An item that costs $6.00 sells for $9.99. What percent profit is made on each sale of the item?
    a) 39.9%
    b) 66.5%
    c) 16%
    d) 3.9%

51. Which of the following medications is not an antihistamine?
    a) Chlorpheniramine
    b) Diphenhydramine
    c) Hydroxyzine
    d) Benzonatate

52. Dextromethorphan is an antitussive agent included in many cough preparations.
    a) True
    b) False

53. An item that currently retails for $79.99 cost the pharmacy only $50.00. What is the profit margin on each sale of this item?
    a) 62.5%
    b) 60%
    c) 48%
    d) 37.5%

54. Oxygen passes through the thin alveolus wall to the hemoglobin of red blood cells.
    a) True
    b) False

55. Which of the following medications is an antihistamine?
    a) Cephalexin
    b) Tolteradine
    c) Hydroxyzine
    d) Lisdexamfetamine

56. _____ are used to reduce the itch, flare and wheal response the body often has with an allergic reaction.
    a) Antihistamines
    b) Expectorants
    c) Nasal Decongestants
    d) Bronchodilators

57. A patient who's been diagnosed with shingles has been prescribed an antiviral. Which of the following meds may have been written for that patient?
    a) Lyrica
    b) Detrol LA
    c) Abilify
    d) Valtrex

58. Strips for a glucometer sell for $54.39 per package. The actual cost of the strips is $42.00. What percent profit is made on this product?
    a) 22.8%
    b) 29.5%
    c) 46.7%
    d) 77.2%

59. _____ are indicated for a non-productive cough with a presence of mucous in the respiratory tract.
    a) Antitussives
    b) Antihistamines
    c) Expectorants
    d) Bronchodilators

60. The boss wishes to earn a 24% profit on an item that costs $14.20. What would the dollar value of the markup need to be to ensure this amount of profit?
    a) $17.61
    b) $10.79
    c) $6.82
    d) $3.41

61. Antihistamines reduce the amount of mucous secretions and cause a drying effect.
    a) True   b) False

62. The pharmacy plans to make 40% profit margin on an item that costs just $3.80. What is the necessary retail price amount for such a profit?
    a) $1.52   c) $5.32
    b) $2.28   d) $6.26

63. Flonase is an inhaled corticosteroid medication.
    a) True   b) False

64. Which of the following is a bronchodilator?
    a) Flunisolide   d) Both a and b
    b) Albuterol   e) Both b and c
    c) Theophylline   f) Both a and c

65. The drug Singulair carries a primary indication of bronchostriction inhibition.
    a) True   b) False

66. The retail price of a ankle brace is $12.69 The acquisition cost of the brace is only $7.40 What percent profit is being made on the sale of the brace?
    a) 28.3%   c) 58.3%
    b) 41.7%   d) 71.5%

67. Indocin and Mobic are both classed as a(n)_____ drugs.
    a) antibacterial   c) antipsychotic
    b) NSAID   d) antiviral

68. Beclomethasone is known as a nasal decongestant.
    a) True   b) False

69. The entire gas exchange process is referred to as _____.
    a) External respiration   c) Blood filtering
    b) Internal respiration   d) None of these

70. _____ dilate the bronchioles to reverse bronchospasms.
    a) Leukotriene receptor antagonists   c) Decongestants
    b) Antihistamines   d) None of these

71. Taking meloxicam can place patients at an increased risk of _____.
    a) tendonitis   c) serious cardiovascular events
    b) suicidal thoughts   d) infection

72. As blood passes through the lungs and nears the thin aveolus walls, carbon dioxide is passed from the blood where it can be exhaled.
    a) True   b) False

73. The total charge of a sale is $11.28. The customer pays with a twenty dollar bill. What is the value of the returned change?
   a) $3.72
   b) $8.72
   c) $28.72
   d) $8.28

74. Which of the following are inhaled corticosteroids?
   a) Flovent
   b) Azmacort
   c) Pulmicort
   d) Both a and b
   e) Both b and c
   f) All of these

75. The law that requires pseudoephedrine products behind the counter for purchasing is commonly called _____.
   a) FDA Modernization Act
   b) Poison Prevention Act
   c) Combat Meth Act
   d) None of these

76. Ipratropium is a bronchodilator.
   a) True
   b) False

Match the following drugs to their generic names.

77. Keflex   _____ a) tolterodine
78. Coreg   _____ b) hydroxyzine
79. Lanoxin   _____ c) indomethacin
80. Lyrica   _____ d) valacyclovir
81. Abilify   _____ e) meloxicam
82. Mobic   _____ f) cefdinir
83. Indocin   _____ g) lisdexamfetamine
84. Valtrex   _____ h) aripiprazole
85. Vyvanse   _____ i) pregabalin
86. Omnicef   _____ j) digoxin
87. Vistaril   _____ k) carvedilol
88. Detrol LA   _____ l) cephalexin

Match the following drugs to their classifications.

89. Digoxin   _____ a) cephalosporin
90. Carvedilol   _____ b) antimuscarinic
91. Cephalexin   _____ c) beta-blocker
92. Hydroxyzine   _____ d) antihistamine
93. Tolterodine   _____ e) CNS stimulant
94. Indomethacin   _____ f) NSAID
95. Pregabalin   _____ g) cardiac glycoside
96. Cefdinir   _____ h) NSAID
97. Valacyclovir   _____ i) antiviral
98. Meloxicam   _____ j) antipsychotic
99. Lisdexamfetamine   _____ k) anticonvulsant
100. Aripiprazole   _____ l) cephalosporin

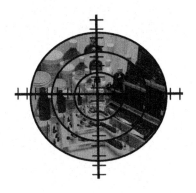

Mission 13
Infections and
Therapeutic Treatments

Mission Objectives

*To understand the various types of infections.

*To learn of the drug families used in treating infections.

*To understand the pharmacology of drugs used in infections.

*To gain baseline knowledge of twelve popular drugs on the market.

*To review all types of general pharmacy calculations.

Infections are formed from a disease-causing organism's invasion on the body. It could be a bacterial, viral, fungal, or parasitic invasion. Everyone carries germs or microorganisms but most of the time, the body defends itself against an invasion. As studied in Mission 11, the white blood cells or leukocytes are the body's defense against infection. Occasionally and for a variety of reasons these microorganisms get passed the body's standard defense mechanisms and try to set up a homestead.

Most invaders that are **bacterial**, such as streptococci, staphylococci, bacilli and spirilla cause infections that can normally be treated with antibiotic therapy. Depending on the resistance or susceptibility, different classes of antibiotics are available. **Antibiotic resistance** is becoming more prominent as time progresses. Reasons for this resistance vary from patients' non-compliance to complete the regimen of antibiotic medications prescribed by their physicians to the increased use of antibacterial cleansers and many other factors.

Viruses are much smaller than bacteria and usually do not respond well or at all to antibiotics. In fact, if an antibacterial is prescribed to a patient having a virus, it is most often done to prevent or treat a secondary infection. Most viruses such as the common cold just have to run "their course" and if strong enough, the body will eventually rid itself of the invader. Other more serious viruses benefit from the new antiviral medications that are now available within the last decade. Many of these drugs were developed to help patients with chronic viral infections.

Fungi are plant-like microorganisms that cause various health problems ranging from ringworm to candidiasis, which is commonly referred to as a yeast infection. Antifungal medications are available in oral, topical, and even intravenous dosage forms.

It is a proven fact that bacteria which are not killed during antibiotic treatment or disinfecting of areas where germs are harbored are able to mutate and become stronger and more resilient to the current treatments that are available.

Parasitic infections occur when small organisms like lice, worms or other protozoa attach themselves to the body or enter the body in some way and begin to feed off the host. There are topical and oral preparations that are indicated for treatment of such invasions. Most parasites and protozoa cannot live for very long without being attached to or inside a host's body.

Proper hygiene is the key to help prevent the spreading of many diseases. Proper **hand washing** is the number one defense mechanism against the spread of infection. There are many ways that infection is spread, but direct contact is the most probable way disease is passed from one to another. Other ways include, airborne and blood borne pathogens. The airborne bacteria can be passed from one person to another unknowingly. Blood borne pathogens must have blood or body fluids contact before they can be passed from one source to another.

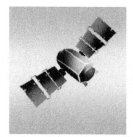

Recon Mission 13:

With this mission's reconnaissance you are encouraged to search the Internet for information on various types of infections. Write down as many of the conditions as you can find with a brief description of each one. As you continue on this mission, some medications may be discussed that are used primarily to treat diseases and disorders that you have read about and familiarized yourself with. You are encouraged to devote plenty of time to this activity. In addition, there are two major organizations that work very hard to keep the public domain informed of information concerning infections and how to be protected.

* The **Centers for Disease Control and Prevention** – a government organization which provides health and safety information regarding infections, epidemics and many other topics surrounding public safety. www.cdc.gov

* The **World Health Organization** is the leading authority on health matters within the United Nations system. They provide leadership on health matters from a world standpoint. www.who.int

Therapeutic Treatments

Penicillin is the oldest form of antibiotic therapy. There are many variations and several combinations of penicillamines available for use. Most of the antibiotics containing penicillin should be given on an empty stomach or without regard to meals for the best absorption and results available. Solme drugs in this class are quite probable to cause GI upset and generally those are recommended to be taken with food. Those penicillin injectable products that are ready to use, such as Penicillin G, must be refrigerated to until use to preserve stability. In addition, ampicillin injection should be mixed with sodium chloride for **best** stability, though it can be diluted in other fluids.

* Pen Vee K – Penicillin V Potassium
* Amoxil – Amoxicillin
* Dynapen – Dicloxacillin
* Totacillin – Ampicillin
* Augmentin-Amoxicillin/Potassium Clavulanate
* Piperacil - Piperacillin
* BiCillin LA - Penicillin G

Cephalosporins were the next generation of antibiotic treatment that became available. Since the first generation of cephalosporins were marketed there have been numerous additions to this family of antibacterials. The absorption of this class of medications is delayed by food but not necessarily changed. The medications in this class, like the penicillins, are generally very broad spectrum. This means that various strains of bacteria will be sensitive to them.

* Keflex – Cephalexin
* Duricef – Cefadroxil
* Cefzil – Cefprozil
* Rocephin – Ceftriaxone
* Ancef – Cefazolin
* Claforan – Cefotaxime

Many patients have an allergy to penicillin. If a patient is allergic to penicillin, there is a ten percent chance that they will also be allergic to cephalasporins. This is what is known as **cross-sensitivity**.

Fluoroquinolones are a newer class of antibiotic therapy. This class of drugs is still relatively broad-spectrum therapy. One of the advantages of taking fluoroquinolones, as opposed to the afore mentioned classes of drugs is that a more convenient dosing regimen is allowed. Where the penicillins and cephalosporins are dosed three or four times daily, a fluoroquinolone would only need to be taken once or twice daily. Though food may delay absorption, most of the drugs in this class can be given without regard to meals.

Generally, the quinolone family of antibiotics is not used in children under the age of 18. However, some cases of severe infection may justify their use in this age group.

* Cipro – Ciprofloxacin
* Floxin – Ofloxacin
* Levaquin – Levofloxacin
* Avelox – Moxifloxacin

Macrolides also offer newer opportunities to treat bacterial infections. Although the drug of choice in treating a streptococcal infection has always been the penicillin derivatives, for those allergic to penicillins, macrolides offer an effective alternative. Convenient dosing is likely to be a top advantage for using a medication from the macrolide class. Dosing is generally once or twice a day depending on the medication and the infection being treated.

* Biaxin – Clarithromycin
* Zithromax – Azithromycin
* Ery-Tab – Erythromycin

We see **tetracyclines** used to treat skin problems such as acne more so than other classes of antibiotic therapy. Although there are other indications for this class of medications, this is one of their primary uses in today's world of pharmacy. When taking tetracyclines, patients should avoid dairy products and antacids because the medicine will bind to the dairy products or antacids, while in the gut, and will not be absorbed. In addition, this class of therapeutic treatment can cause severe photosensitivity so patients should avoid or limit sunlight exposure during treatment. Auxiliary labels are generally affixed to the dispensing label with these instructions to help warn patients of these situations.

* Sumycin – Tetracycline
* Vibratab – Doxycycline
* Minocin – Minocycline

Some other **Miscellaneous antibiotics/antibacterials** are listed below. Those patients who are allergic to sulpha drugs should avoid the use of sulfamethoxazole/trimethoprim. Those patients taking the drug metronidazole should avoid the use of alcohol during therapy. It will cause an emetic type action similar to that of Antabuse and will make the patient very sick.

* Bactrim –Sulfamethoxazole/ Trimethoprim
* Macrodantin – Nitrofurantoin
* Flagyl – Metronidazole

Amphotericin B must be stored under refrigeration and should be diluted or mixed with dextrose for stability purposes.

Antifungal agents are used to treat such conditions as candidiasis, which is found in vaginal yeast infections, some diaper rashes, and thrush in infants. Ringworm, jock itch and athlete's foot are also fungal infections that need an antifungal agent for treatment. Some of the newest fungal treatments being used are that of agents given to treat nail fungus. Medications in this class are available in topical, oral and injectable forms.

* Grifulvin – Griseofulvin
* Mycostatin – Nystatin
* Diflucan – Fluconazole
* Sporanox   – Itraconazole
* Lamisil – Terbinafine
* Fungizone   – Amphotericin B

Tuberculosis is an airborne lung disease that is highly contagious. At this time, there is no known cure for TB and healthcare organizations are required to test employees annually for TB. Sometimes after exposure to this disease, a person will have a positive skin test for TB. This does not necessarily mean that that person has TB per say, but the person will be a carrier and must be given prophylaxis treatment so as not to develop TB. This includes a bi-weekly regimen of a combination of drug therapy. Some of the TB meds are listed below.
* INH – Isoniazide
* Rifadin -Rifampin
* Myambutol – Ethambutol
* Vitamin B_6 –Pyridoxine

Antiviral agents are primarily used to treat such conditions as HIV and herpes. Up until the last few years, most patients infected with the HIV virus developed full blown AIDS as time passed. With the updated treatment available through new medications, more and more patients are able to live longer and with fewer complications. With genital herpes, medications can be taken at maintenance doses to prevent outbreaks and at increased doses during the time of an outbreak. These medications can also be used to treat other forms of the herpes simplex virus such as chickenpox, severe fever blisters and shingles.
* Zovirax – Acyclovir
* Famvir – Famciclovir
* Crixivan – Indinavir
* Viracept – Nelfinavir
* Valtrex– Valacyclovir

Influenza, commonly called the "flu", is also a member of the virus family. The best protection from contracting the influenza virus is to receive the "flu" vaccine on an annual basis. However, there are special medications that can be used to treat this virus that vary from the other antiviral medications. Most of these options are only effective if used within the first 24 to 48 hours of infection. Relenza is a newer version of flu treatment. It comes in the form of a powdered inhalant. Others are available in an oral form. With the flu virus, if these medications are not effective, the patient can still receive some relief by symptomatic treatment with other medications, most of which are over the counter.
* Flumadine – Rimantadine
* Symmetrel – Amantadine
* Relenza – Zanamivir
* Tamiflu – Oseltamivir

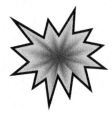

Math Blaster

For the Mission 13 Math Blaster, feel free to review the explanations in previous missions for the pharmacy calculations. In the mission 13 debriefing, you will be revisiting the skills learned in all of the earlier Missions.

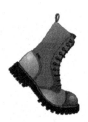

Drill Practice

For this mission's drill practice, rework any sections of math that you still seem to have difficulty. In the Mission 13 debriefing, you will be checking to see how well you remember all of your skills.

Drug Training Chapter Thirteen

Brand Name	Generic Name	Drug Classification	Primary Indication	Side effects, Warnings, Other
Spiriva	Tiotropium	Inhaled Bronchodilator	COPD, chronic bronchitis and emphysema	Dry mouth, constipation or trouble with urination
Atripla	Efavirenz, emtricitabine, and tenofovir	Antiviral	HIV	lactic acidosis, hepatotoxicity, depression, osteopenia dizziness, headache, insomnia or drowsiness, trouble concentrating, unusual dreams
Stendra	Avanafil	ED agent	Erectile Dysfunction	headache, flushing, nasal congestion and other cold-like symptoms and back pain
Celebrex	celecoxib	NSAID cox-2 inhibitor	osteoarthritis, rheumatoid arthritis, spondylitis, acute pain, dysmenorrhea	increased risk of serious cardiovascular thrombotic events, myocardial infarction, and stroke, gi bleeding, ulceration, and perforation of the stomach or intestines which can be fatal.
Provigil	Modafinil	C IV Narcoleptic agent	Excessive sleepiness, sleep apnea and other sleep disorders	Rash, persistent sleepiness, Suicidal ideation, aggression
Premarin	Conjugated Estrogens	Sex Hormone	Hormone replacement therapy in post-menopausal woment	May increase risk of breast and endometrial cancer, stroke, blood clots; may also cause arthralgia, myalgia, leg cramps, breast tenderness/enlargement
Ventolin HFA	albuterol	Inhaled bronchodilator	treatment or prevention of bronchospasm	Throat irritation, upper respiratory inflammation, viral respiratory infections, cough, musculoskelatal pain

Brand Name	Generic Name	Drug Classification	Primary Indication	Side effects, Warnings, Other
Diovan	Valsartan	angiotensin II receptor blocker (ARB)	hypertension	Contraindicated in pregnancy,
Arimidex	Anastrozole	Aromatase inhibitors	Breast cancer in post menopausal women	hot flashes, arthralgia, weakness, mood changes, pain, sore throat, nausea/ vomiting rash, depression, hypertension, osteoporosis, insomnia, headache.
Prograf	Tacrolimus	Immunosuppressive agents	Antirejection for transplant patients	Increased susceptibility to infections, back pain, tremors, Confusion, numbness or tingling
Strattera	Atomoxetine	CNS stimulants	Attention Deficit Hyperactivity Disorder	Possible increase in suicidal thoughts, depression, mood swings or changes
Mirapex	Pramipexole	Dopaminergic antiparkinsonism agents	Parkinson's Disease Restless Leg Syndrome	Nausea, headaches, insomnia or drowsiness, weakness, tics, hypotension, abnormal dreams

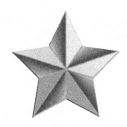

Mission 13 Debriefing

Answer the following questions in assessment of the lessons learned in Mission 13. For best results, repeat the exercise until no questions are missed.

1. Tetracycline may cause the side effect of photosensitivity.
   a) True
   b) False

2. If a pharmacy pricing formula is the average wholesale price (AWP) plus $4.50 and the AWP is $90 for 100 tablets, what is the charge for a prescription for 30 tablets?
   a) $27.00
   b) $30.50
   c) $31.50
   d) $13.50

3. Which of the following are different types of infections?
   a) Bacterial
   b) Fungal
   c) Viral
   d) Parasitic
   e) Only a and c
   f) Only b and c
   g) Only b and d
   h) All of these are infections

4. Taking the drug celecoxib places patients at a higher risk of suffering _____.
   a) tendonitis
   b) serious cardiovascular events
   c) breast or endometrial cancer
   d) infections

5. Most parasites, worms or protozoa cannot live for very long without a host from which they gain nourishment.
   a) True
   b) False

6. Patients who are allergic to penicillin have a 1:10 probability of also being allergic to _____.
   a) Fluoroquinolones
   b) Cephalosporins
   c) Macrolides
   d) None of these

7. How many 500 mg doses can be prepared from a 10 g vial of cefazolin?
   a) 50 doses
   b) 2 doses
   c) 10 doses
   d) 20 doses

8. Which of the following pairs of medications are inhaled bronchodilators?
   a) Provigil and Premarin
   b) Spiriva and Ventolin HFA
   c) Strattera and Stendra
   d) Arimadex and Atripla

9. Cross-sensitivity means an allergy to one substance could mean an allergy to another.
   a) True
   b) False

10. Which of the following is classed as a fluoroquinolone antibiotic?
    a) Zithromax
    b) Levaquin
    c) Vibratab
    d) All of these

11. The technician receives an order for KCL 40meq/1000mL NS to be infused at 80mL/hr. What amount of KCL will the patient receive per hour?
    a) 3.2mEq
    b) 12.5mEq
    c) 32mEq
    d) 48mEq

12. Ampicillin injections should be mixed or diluted with dextrose solution for best stability
    a) True
    b) False

13. Streptococci is a _____ and will typically respond to susceptible therapy.
    a) Virus
    b) Parasite
    c) Fungus
    d) Bacteria

14. HIV patients are able to live longer and with fewer complications than in years past because better medications and treatments are available.
    a) True
    b) False

15. Stendra is classified as a(n) _____.
    a) Bronchodilator
    b) Erectile dysfunction agent
    c) Aromatase inhibitor
    d) Immunosupressant

16. Antifungal medications can be found in which dosage forms?
    a) Topical
    b) Oral
    c) Injectable
    d) All of these

17. An IV infusion order is written for 1000mL of $D_5W/0.45\%NS$ to run over 12 hours. The set you have will deliver 15gtts/mL. What should the flow rate be in gtts/min?
    a) 83gtts/min
    b) 63gtts/min
    c) 21gtts/min
    d) 10gtts/min

18. Which of the following medications is not classed with the penicillins?
    a) Augmentin
    b) Claforan
    c) Amoxil
    d) Piperacil

19. Tuberculosis is a highly contagious disease transmitted through blood born pathogens.
    a) True
    b) False

20. _____ is the best defense against the spread of infection.
    a) Wearing gloves
    b) Washing hands
    c) Wiping front counters
    d) Taking antibiotics

21. If a patient has been prescribed an NSAID, which of these medications could have been written on the prescription?
    a) Avanafil
    b) Celecoxib
    c) Modafanil
    d) Pramipexole

22. Which class includes many broad spectrum antibiotics?
    a) Penicillins
    b) Cephalosporins
    c) Both a and b
    d) Neither a nor b

23. How many 1 liter bags (1000mL) will be needed if a patient is getting Normal Saline continuous infusion at a rate of 125mL/hr for 24 hours?
    a) 1 bag
    b) 2 bags
    c) 3 bags
    d) 4 bags

24. Which of the following is a cephalosporin antibacterial agent?
    a) Keflex
    b) Duricef
    c) Rocephin
    d) All of these

25. Viruses are _____ than bacteria and treating them usually does not include antibiotic therapy.
    a) larger
    b) smaller
    c) neither, they are same size

26. A patient who takes the drug Atripla probably has been diagnosed with _____.
    a) HIV
    b) ED
    c) Asthma
    d) Narcolepsy

27. Tamiflu is an inhaled form of therapy used to treat the influenza virus.
    a) True
    b) False

28. A dermatologist frequently orders 2 oz of the following prescription:
    LCD 2% Salicylic acid 5% QSAD yellow petrolatum. The pharmacy technician wants to prepare a 500 g bulk amount, and then prepackage it in 2 oz containers. How much salicylic acid will be needed to compound the 500 g?
    a) 10g
    b) 25g
    c) 8g
    d) 14g

29. Modafinil is a _____ controlled substance.
    a) C II
    b) C III
    c) C IV
    d) C V

30. Amphotericin B should be mixed with sodium chloride for best stability.
    a) True
    b) False

31. Patients may prefer the use of _____ because they are available with more convenient dosing regimens.
    a) Fluoroquinolones
    b) Macrolides
    c) Both a and b
    d) Neither a nor b

32. A child should receive Tegretol at 20mg/kg/day in 3 equal doses. If the patient weighs 38lbs what will be the strength of each dose?
    a) 17mg
    b) 115mg
    c) 173mg
    d) 346mg

33. Strattera is a _____ controlled substance.
    a) C II
    b) C III
    c) C IV
    d) C V
    e) None of these

34. Which of the following might a TB patient be prescribed?
    a) Isoniazide
    b) Valcyclovir
    c) Nystatin
    d) Griseofulvin

35. Ringworm is a type of fungal infection.
    a) True
    b) False

36. Determine the flow rate in mL/hr if 50mL of mannitol is to be administered over a 2 hour period and the set delivers 60gtts/mL.
    a) 25mL/hr
    b) 20mL/hr
    c) 15mL/hr
    d) 4 0mL/hr

37. Valsartan is indicated for _____.
    a) Parkinsonism
    b) Breast cancer
    c) Narcolepsy
    d) Hypertension

38. A patient gives the pharmacy a prescription for Cephalexin 250mg, ii po tid x7. How many capsules will be needed to fill the order?
    a) 21
    b) 30
    c) 42
    d) 56

39. Ethambutol is indicated to treat patients with _____.
    a) A bacterial infection
    b) Tuberculosis
    c) Shingles
    d) Acne

40. Arimedex is an agent for patients with erectile dysfunction.
    a) True
    b) False

41. A patient who's had a kidney transplant is likely to be taking which of the following medications?
    a) Atomoxetine
    b) Tacrolimus
    c) Pramipexole
    d) Effavirenz

42. Current medication therapies offer patients with genital herpes treatment plans for maintenance dosing to prevent outbreaks as well as increased dosing regimens during those times when outbreaks occur.
   a) True   b) False

43. The best protection against contracting the influenza virus is_____.
   a) hand washing   c) annual vaccine
   b) personal hygiene   d) isolation

44. Levaquin is classified as a broad spectrum Macrolide antibiotic.
   a) True   b) False

45. Healthcare workers are generally tested _____ for tuberculosis.
   a) every 5 years   c) biannually
   b) every 3 years   d) annually

46. A patient brings the following script to your pharmacy: Amoxicillin 400mg po tid for 10 days. You have in stock Amoxicillin 250mg/5mL. What is the exact volume of medication you will need for filling this script?
   a) 240mL   c) 300mL
   b) 180mL   d) 320mL

47. Patients who take Strattera have an increased risk of suicidal thoughts.
   a) True   b) False

48. Which of these groups is the oldest form of antibiotic therapy?
   a) Cephalosporins   c) Macrolids
   b) Penicillins   d) Fluoroquinolones

49. The following order is written: prednisolone liquid, 1tsp tid x2 days, then 1 tsp bid x2 days, then 1 tsp qd x2 days. How much prednisolone will be needed to fill the order?
   a) 70mL   c) 40mL
   b) 35mL   d) 60mL

50. Doxycycline should be taken with milk for best absorption.
   a) True   b) False

51. Which of the following could contribute to antibiotic resistance?
   a) Overuse of antibiotics   c) Increased use of antibacterial cleansers
   b) Noncompliance with antibiotic use   d) All of these

52. A patient may increase their risk of succumbing to breast or endometrial cancer if they are prescribed _____.
   a) Provigil   c) Premarin
   b) Stendra   d) Prograf

53. Oseltamivir is primarily indicated for patients who have "the flu".
   a) True   b) False

54. A patient with an allergy to sulpha products should avoid which of these medications.
    a) Keflex
    b) Amoxil
    c) Levaquin
    d) Bactrim

55. Which of the following are treated with antifungal agents?
    a) Yeast infections
    b) Ringworm
    c) Nail fungus
    d) All of these

56. Where should injectable ready-to-use pencillin products such as Penicillin G be stored?
    a) On the pharmacy shelf at room temperature
    b) In the refrigerator
    c) In a locked cabinet for controlled substances
    d) In the freezer area of the refrigerator

57. Alcohol use should be avoided when taking metronidazole.
    a) True
    b) False

58. Candidiasis is another word for the commonly known_____.
    a) chronic cough
    b) athlete's foot
    c) yeast infection
    d) jock itch

59. Macrolides offer an excellent treatment alternative in patients with streptococcal infection who are allergic to penicillin products.
    a) True
    b) False

60. A patient in the hospital needs KCl 8meq IV stat. You have in stock KCl 20meq/mL in a 10mL Multi Dose Vial. What will the volume of the stat dose be?
    a) 2.5mL
    b) 0.4mL
    c) 4mL
    d) 1.6mL

61. The drug Mirapex has an indication for _____.
    a) breast cancer treatment
    b) hypertension
    c) restless leg syndrome
    d) depression

62. A patient taking Prograf is at an increased risk of _____.
    a) suicidal thoughts
    b) endometrial cancer
    c) heart attack
    d) infections

63. Which of the following are ways that infections might be transmitted?
    a) Blood borne pathogens
    b) Direct contact
    c) Airborne particles
    d) All of these

64. Influenza or "the flu" is a bacterial infection and can be treated with antibiotic therapy.
    a) True
    b) False

65. _____ infections occur when small organisms attach themselves to or enter the body of their host to feed.
    a) Viral
    b) Parasitic
    c) Fungal
    d) Bacterial

66. Generally, which class of antibiotics are not recommended for children under 18 unless the situation is extreme and the infection is severe.
    a) Penicillins
    b) Fluoroquinolones
    c) Cephalosporins
    d) Macrolides

67. Using alcohol products while taking metronidazole can cause a severe emetic reaction.
    a) True
    b) False

68. Various antiviral medications are used to treat which of the following conditions?
    a) Chickenpox
    b) Influenza
    c) Genital herpes
    d) HIV patients
    e) Shingles
    f) Only b and d
    g) Only c and d
    h) All of these are treated with antivirals

69. Minocin ,a tetracycline derivative antibacterial, should not be taken with milk or antacids.
    a) True
    b) False

70. Tuberculosis agents include all but which of the following?
    a) Vitamin B6
    b) INH
    c) Rifadian
    d) All of these

71. Which of the following is not a macrolide antibacterial agent?
    a) Floxin
    b) Biaxin
    c) Zithromax
    d) Erytab

72. _____ is the generic name for Sporanox.
    a) Griseofulvin
    b) Fluconazole
    c) Terbinafine
    d) Itraconazole

73. All but which of the following are antiviral agents?
    a) Zithromax
    b) Crixivan
    c) Valtrex
    d) Viracept

74. The CDC is the leading authority on infection control within the United Nations.
    a) True
    b) False

75. Blood borne pathogens must have direct contact with _____ before they can be passed from one source to another.
    a) Blood or blood products
    b) Body fluids
    c) Either a or b
    d) Neither a nor b

76. Which of these cells help to defend against infection by attacking and destroying bacteria and other microorganisms?
    a) Red blood cells
    b) White blood cells
    c) Platelets
    d) None of these

Match the following drugs to their generic names.

77. Spiriva
78. Diovan
79. Ventolin HFA
80. Mirapex
81. Atripla
82. Arimidex
83. Premarin
84. Strattera
85. Stendra
86. Provigil
87. Prograf
88. Celebrex

_____ a) pramipexole
_____ b) atomoxetine
_____ c) tacrolimus
_____ d) anastrozole
_____ e) valsartan
_____ f) albuterol
_____ g) conjugated estrogens
_____ h) modafinil
_____ i) celecoxib
_____ j) avanafil
_____ k) efavirenz/emtricitabine/tenofovir
_____ l) tiotropium

Match the following drugs to their classifications.

89. Atomoxetine
90. Valsartan
91. Anastrozole
92. Tacrolimus
93. Pramipexole
94. Modafinil
95. Avanafil
96. Celecoxib
97. Albuterol
98. Tiotropium
99. Conjugated estrogens
100. Efavirenze/emtricitabine Tenofovir combination

_____ a) inhaled bronchodilator
_____ b) antiviral
_____ c) sex hormone
_____ d) narcoleptic agent
_____ e) ED agent
_____ f) NSAID
_____ g) angiotensin receptor blocker (ARB)
_____ h) aromatase inhibitor
_____ i) CNS stimulant
_____ j) dopaminergic/antiparkinsonism agent
_____ k) inhaled bronchodilator
_____ l) imminunosppressive agent

Answers to Drill Practice Mission 1

1. 1
2. 4
3. 6
4. 8
5. 6.9
6. 3.5
7. 2.1
8. 78.4
9. 71.25
10. 2.68
11. 58.68
12. 101.1
13. 25.643
14. 218.869
15. 1049.031
16. 12.007
17. 32%
18. 74%
19. 8%
20. 81%
21. 40%
22. 2.5%
23. 80%
24. 4.75%
25. 0.96
26. 0.0327
27. 0.478
28. 0.56
29. 0.02
30. 0.008
31. 0.74
32. 0.0287

Answers to Drill Practice Mission 2

1. 30
2. 12
3. 9
4. 90
5. 60
6. 14
7. 1000
8. 42
9. XX
10. XXVIII
11. XL
12. X
13. VII
14. XV
15. XVI
16. VIII

Ratio	Fraction	Decimal	Percent
3:3	$\frac{3}{4}$	0.75	75 %
3:5	$\frac{3}{5}$	0.6	60%
63:100	$\frac{63}{100}$	0.63	63%
2:3	$\frac{2}{3}$	0.67	67%
21:50	$\frac{21}{50}$	0.42	42%
7:8	$\frac{7}{8}$	0.875	87.5%
9:25	$\frac{9}{25}$	0.36	36%
1:8	$\frac{1}{8}$	0.125	12.5%
1:25	$\frac{1}{25}$	0.04	4%
1:4	$\frac{1}{4}$	0.25	25%

Answers to Drill Practice Mission 3

1. 2mL
2. 15mEq
3. 8mL
4. 120 tabs
5. 630mL
6. 5 patches
7. 315mL
8. 36 tabs
9. 7 days supply
10. 7 days supply
11. 4 days
12. 2 vials – 17 days
13. 4 vials – 8 days
14. C
15. C
16. 240mL
17. 112mL
18. 3mL, 42mL
19. 16 doses
20. 25 doses

Answers to Drill Practice Mission 4

1. 1.35mL
2. 875mg
3. 100mg
4. 6.4mL
5. 0.5mL
6. 106mg
7. 2.4mL
8. 409-818mg
9. 4500-6000mg
10. 6.25mL
11. 0.25mL
12. 150mg
13. 3000mg or 3g
14. 1.6mL
15. 45-60mg
16. 1.5mL
17. 1.3mL
18. 26-80mg
19. 11.36mg
20. 30mL

Answers to Drill Practice Mission 5

1. 21gtts/min
2. 94mL/hr
3. 25gtts/min
4. 167mL/hr
5. 1920mL
6. 3 bags
7. 71mL/hr
8. 2 bags
9. 42gtts/min
10. 83mL/hr
11. 17gtts/min
12. 63mL/hr
13. 83gtts/min
14. 750mL
15. 2 bags
16. 48gtts/min
17. 2 bags
18. 63mL/hr
19. 125mL/hr
20. 21gtts/min

Answers to Drill Practice Mission 6

1. 10% 151.3g 1% 302.7g
2. 500mL each
3. 10% 108mL water 252mL
4. 2% 150g
5. 6% 320mL water 160mL
6. 120g
7. 0.012g or 120mg since such small amount
8. 2.4%
9. 0.3g or 300mg since such small amount
10. 250g
11. 4%
12. 0.02%
13. 3.75%
14. 6mL
15. 200mL
16. 2.5% 8.3g 1% 16.7g
17. 20%
18. 180g
19. 10% 48mL Hydrophor 72mL
20. 1.5%

Answers to Drill Practice Mission 7

1. 36%
2. 25%
3. 54%
4. 18%
5. 25%
6. $5.06 Mark-up $21.92 selling price
7. $2.43 Mark-up $14.60 selling price
8. $4.19 selling price
9. $30.35 selling price
10. $1.97 Mark-up $ 5.26 selling price
11. $7.00
12. $4.99
13. $22.77
14. $19.80
15. $102.00
16. $20.99
17. $41.39
18. $11.70
19. $6.50
20. $37.49
21. $7.83, 3 pennies, 1 nickel, 3 quarters, 2 dollar bills and 1 five dollar bill
22. $77.85, 1 dime, 3 quarters, 2 dollar bills, 1 five dollar bill, 1 ten dollar bill and 3 twenty dollar bills.
23. $1.38, 3 pennies, 1 dime, 1 quarter, and 1 dollar bill.
24. $19.81, 1 penny, 1 nickel, 3 quarters, 4 one dollar bills, 1 five dollar bill and 1 ten dollar bill.
25. $50.18, 3 pennies, 1 nickel, 1 dime, 1 ten dollar bill and 2 twenties.

Mission 1 Debriefing Answers

1. e	35. b	69. k
2. c	36. b	70. f
3. a	37. b	71. g
4. d	38. a	72. e
5. g	39. d	73. h
6. d	40. a	74. i
7. b	41. b	75. k
8. b	42. b	76. a
9. b and c	43. d	77. g
10. a	44. d	78. b
11. a	45. a	79. d
12. a	46. b	80. f
13. a	47. b	81. c
14. c	48. a	82. h
15. d	49. a	83. e
16. b	50. c	84. j
17. c	51. b	85. l
18. b	52. b	86. 0.8
19. b	53. a	87. 0.2
20. b	54. a	88. 13.19
21. d	55. b	89. 101.29
22. b	56. b	90. 2.087
23. a	57. a	91. 487.052
24. b	58. c	92. 36.899
25. a	59. d	93. 28%
26. c	60. a	94. 1.5%
27. d	61. c	95. 92%
28. a	62. j	96. 41.8%
29. a	63. c	97. 0.495
30. c	64. l	98. 0.321
31. d	65. b	99. 0.00025
32. a	66. i	100. 0.0415
33. a	67. d	
34. b	68. a	

Mission 2 Debriefing Answers

1. AIDS
2. Nausea and vomiting
3. Discharge or discontinue
4. ASAP
5. Date of birth
6. Diagnosis
7. EC
8. I/O
9. Before surgery
10. Long acting
11. CHF
12. STAT
13. TPN
14. US Pharmacopeia
15. Extended release
16. Hx
17. UTI
18. GERD
19. Blood pressure
20. Average wholesale price
21. OTC
22. Blood sugar
23. ICU
24. Post-op
25. After delivery
26. Verbal order
27. HIV
28. EKG (ECG)
29. Bowel movement
30. Prescription Drug Plan
31. K
32. Mg
33. Ca
34. Fe
35. H_2O
36. Na
37. Zn
38. $FeSO_4$
39. $AgNO_3$
40. KCl
41. $CaCO_3$
42. H_2O_2

43. $NaHCO_3$
44. NaCl
45. Kidney
46. Lung
47. Nasal
48. Blood vessel
49. Liver
50. Muscle
51. Bone
52. Anal or Rectal
53. Artery
54. Heart
55. Colon
56. Stomach
57. Lung
58. Skin
59. Vein
60. Ear
61. Cyan
62. Cirrh
63. Erythr
64. Chlor
65. Melan
66. Leuk
67. C
68. F
69. G
70. B
71. D
72. H
73. A
74. E
75. AS
76. PO
77. IM
78. OU
79. SL
80. VAG
81. IV
82. AD
83. PR
84. SQ

85. OS
86. TD
87. AU
88. BUC
89. OD
90. B
91. C
92. B
93. C
94. D
95. C
96. C
97. D
98. B
99. C
100. B
101. A
102. C
103. C
104. A
105. C
106. D
107. A
108. D
109. B
110. G
111. I
112. K
113. A
114. C
115. E
116. H
117. J
118. L
119. B
120. D

121. F
122. K
123. I
124. G
125. E
126. Either C, H, L
127. A
128. Either H, C, L
129. J
130. Either L, H, C
131. F
132. D
133. B
134. 20
135. 11
136. 4
137. 110
138. 54
139. 15
140. 100
141. 44
142. XXX
143. XXIV
144. L
145. XIII
146. IX
147. XVII
148. VI
149. IV

	Ratio	Fraction	Decimal	Percent
150.	1:3	1/3	0.33	33%
151.	2:5	2/5	0.4	40%
152.	23:50	23/50	0.46	46%
153.	5:8	5/8	0.625	62.5%
154.	1:2	1/2	0.5	50%
155.	2:3	2/3	0.67	67%

Mission 3 Debriefing Answers

1. b	35. c	69. 3
2. c	36. d	70. 2
3. c	37. b	71. 3
4. b	38. c	72. 1
5. a	39. a	73. 2
6. b	40. b	74. 3
7. b	41. b	75. 2
8. c	42. a	76. 3
9. b	43. b	77. h
10. a	44. b	78. g
11. d	45. d	79. c
12. a	46. c	80. b
13. b	47. c	81. f
14. c	48. a	82. k
15. a	49. a	83. l
16. c	50. b	84. i
17. b	51. a	85. e
18. b	52. a	86. a
19. d	53. d	87. d
20. d	54. d	88. j
21. a	55. a	89. k
22. a	56. d	90. a
23. b	57. a	91. l
24. b	58. d	92. b
25. c	59. b	93. i
26. d	60. a	94. c
27. c	61. a	95. h
28. a	62. a	96. d (or g)
29. a	63. d	97. f
30. d	64. c	98. j
31. a	65. 1	99. e
32. b	66. 3	100. g (or d)
33. c	67. 3	
34. b	68. 2	

Mission 4 Debriefing Answers

1. c	35. a	69. a
2. b	36. a	70. a
3. a	37. c	71. a
4. c	38. b	72. b
5. b	39. c	73. b
6. c	40. c	74. b
7. a	41. b	75. c
8. f	42. d	76. a
9. b	43. b	77. g
10. b	44. c	78. a
11. c	45. a	79. k
12. d	46. b	80. b
13. d	47. a	81. l
14. a	48. b	82. c
15. a	49. b	83. f
16. a	50. a	84. i
17. a	51. d	85. e
18. a	52. b	86. h
19. b	53. c	87. d
20. b	54. b	88. j
21. a	55. d	89. b (or g)
22. d	56. b	90. l
23. a	57. c	91. e (or j)
24. a	58. b	92. f
25. c	59. d	93. g (or b)
26. a	60. d	94. i
27. b	61. a	95. h
28. b	62. b	96. j (or e)
29. b	63. a	97. c
30. b	64. c	98. k
31. b	65. c	99. d
32. d	66. b	100. a
33. b	67. a	
34. c	68. e	

Mission 5 Debriefing Answers

1.	d	35.	d	69.	f		
2.	b	36.	b	70.	b		
3.	b	37.	b	71.	h		
4.	a	38.	d	72.	j		
5.	b	39.	b	73.	c		
6.	d	40.	b	74.	e		
7.	d	41.	b	75.	i		
8.	d	42.	b	76.	d		
9.	b	43.	d	77.	e		
10.	b	44.	d	78.	a		
11.	b	45.	d	79.	i		
12.	e	46.	a	80.	b		
13.	a	47.	a	81.	l		
14.	a	48.	b	82.	k		
15.	b	49.	c	83.	d		
16.	b	50.	c	84.	c		
17.	c	51.	a	85.	j		
18.	c	52.	b	86.	h		
19.	b	53.	d	87.	f		
20.	a	54.	a	88.	g		
21.	c	55.	c	89.	l		
22.	d	56.	c	90.	k		
23.	a	57.	d	91.	j		
24.	d	58.	d	92.	i		
25.	c	59.	b	93.	h		
26.	d	60.	c	94.	g		
27.	b	61.	a	95.	a		
28.	a	62.	b	96.	b		
29.	b	63.	2	97.	c		
30.	b	64.	1	98.	d		
31.	a	65.	4	99.	e		
32.	b	66.	3	100.	f		
33.	a	67.	g				
34.	b	68.	a				

Mission 6 Debriefing Answers

1. d	35. b	69. d
2. b	36. a	70. b
3. c	37. a	71. 6
4. d	38. b	72. 4
5. b	39. b	73. 1
6. d	40. a	74. 5
7. a	41. c	75. 2
8. a	42. b	76. 3
9. a	43. b	77. e
10. a	44. c	78. l
11. d	45. b	79. a
12. a	46. d	80. d
13. c	47. a	81. j
14. c	48. a	82. c
15. b	49. d	83. k
16. c	50. a	84. i
17. c	51. d	85. f
18. c	52. b	86. b
19. a	53. a	87. g
20. b	54. d	88. h
21. b	55. a	89. l
22. d	56. a	90. j
23. a	57. b	91. h
24. b	58. b	92. g
25. a	59. d	93. d
26. b	60. a	94. b
27. c	61. a	95. a
28. b	62. c	96. k
29. a	63. a	97. i
30. b	64. a	98. f
31. a	65. c	99. c
32. c	66. b	100. e
33. a	67. d	
34. d	68. a	

Mission 7 Debriefing Answers

1. d	35. d	69. d
2. a	36. d	70. b
3. a	37. c	71. b
4. c	38. a	72. d
5. d	39. e	73. d
6. a	40. b	74. c
7. d	41. b	75. d
8. b	42. b	76. b
9. g	43. b	77. a
10. a	44. c	78. g
11. a	45. a	79. e
12. b	46. f	80. j
13. b	47. b	81. l
14. b	48. a	82. d
15. a	49. c	83. c
16. b	50. b	84. k
17. a	51. d	85. b
18. d	52. b	86. h
19. b	53. a	87. i
20. a	54. d	88. f
21. b	55. b	89. l
22. a	56. d	90. h
23. d	57. a	91. b
24. a	58. d	92. f
25. a	59. a	93. d or g
26. d	60. c	94. k
27. b	61. c	95. g or d
28. a	62. a	96. e
29. b	63. b	97. i
30. d	64. b	98. c
31. b	65. d	99. j
32. b	66. d	100. a
33. c	67. b	
34. a	68. c	

Mission 8 Debriefing Answers

1. b	35. a	69. a
2. d	36. c	70. d
3. d	37. b	71. a
4. d	38. c	72. c
5. a	39. e	73. d
6. a	40. d	74. c
7. d	41. c	75. e
8. c	42. a	76. a
9. a	43. b	77. f
10. c	44. b	78. c
11. a	45. a	79. a
12. b	46. d	80. b
13. d	47. a	81. e
14. b	48. b	82. k
15. b	49. c	83. i
16. a	50. d	84. j
17. a	51. b	85. h
18. d	52. c	86. l
19. a	53. d	87. g
20. c	54. a	88. d
21. b	55. c	89. a or g
22. b	56. d	90. h
23. d	57. b	91. e
24. a	58. c	92. g or a
25. b	59. d	93. b
26. a	60. b	94. f
27. a	61. b	95. d
28. a	62. c	96. l
29. c	63. d	97. i
30. a	64. b	98. j
31. d	65. b	99. c
32. f	66. c	100. k
33. b	67. c	
34. c	68. a	

Mission 9 Debriefing Answers

1. d	35. a	69. b
2. c	36. d	70. c
3. c	37. d	71. c
4. b	38. d	72. b
5. d	39. b	73. b
6. a	40. a	74. c
7. f	41. a	75. d
8. b	42. a	76. b
9. c	43. c	77. d
10. a	44. a	78. a
11. d	45. d	79. c
12. d	46. b	80. j
13. a	47. b	81. l
14. b	48. b	82. i
15. c	49. b	83. f
16. b	50. d	84. k
17. d	51. a	85. b
18. c	52. b	86. e
19. a	53. a	87. g
20. b	54. b	88. h
21. a	55. d	89. g or k
22. c	56. a	90. a
23. b	57. c	91. b or d
24. c	58. a	92. h
25. d	59. b	93. l
26. d	60. c	94. d or b
27. a	61. a	95. f
28. a	62. c	96. j
29. c	63. b	97. c
30. b	64. a	98. i
31. b	65. b	99. k or g
32. a	66. a	100. e
33. b	67. c	
34. a	68. f	

Mission 10 Debriefing Answers

1. d	35. a	69. b
2. a	36. a	70. a
3. b	37. b	71. a
4. c	38. a	72. c
5. b	39. c	73. d
6. c	40. a	74. d
7. f	41. b	75. a
8. b	42. c	76. a
9. d	43. b	77. g
10. b	44. b	78. c
11. c	45. b	79. h
12. c	46. d	80. i
13. a	47. b	81. k
14. d	48. c	82. j
15. a	49. b	83. b
16. b	50. a	84. a
17. b	51. b	85. e
18. d	52. d	86. f
19. c	53. a	87. l
20. d	54. b	88. d
21. a	55. b	89. j
22. b	56. d	90. d
23. b	57. b	91. b
24. a	58. a	92. l
25. f	59. c	93. k
26. c	60. d	94. c
27. a	61. b	95. a
28. b	62. b	96. e
29. a	63. b	97. f
30. c	64. b	98. g
31. a	65. b	99. h
32. d	66. a	100. i
33. a	67. c	
34. d	68. a	

Mission 11 Debriefing Answers

1. b	35. b	69. a
2. b	36. d	70. a
3. d	37. a	71. c
4. b	38. c	72. c
5. b	39. b	73. a
6. b	40. c	74. d
7. c	41. b	75. b
8. a	42. a	76. a
9. c	43. d	77. i
10. b	44. b	78. k
11. d	45. a	79. f
12. a	46. b	80. g
13. b	47. b	81. d
14. d	48. a	82. b
15. f	49. a	83. a
16. b	50. a	84. c
17. b	51. b	85. e
18. b	52. c	86. l
19. a	53. c	87. j
20. c	54. b	88. h
21. b	55. a	89. c
22. d	56. d	90. i
23. b	57. c	91. k
24. c	58. b	92. h
25. b	59. a	93. j
26. a	60. d	94. l
27. c	61. b	95. b
28. a	62. d	96. a
29. d	63. b	97. d
30. a	64. b	98. g
31. c	65. b	99. f
32. b	66. c	100. e
33. b	67. b	
34. d	68. d	

Mission 12 Debriefing Answers

1. b	35. b	69. b
2. d	36. c	70. d
3. a	37. a	71. c
4. a	38. a	72. a
5. b	39. c	73. b
6. b	40. b	74. f
7. d	41. b	75. c
8. b	42. c	76. a
9. b	43. a	77. l
10. d	44. a	78. k
11. a	45. b	79. j
12. c	46. b	80. i
13. d	47. a	81. h
14. a	48. a	82. e
15. c	49. d	83. c
16. b	50. b	84. d
17. c	51. d	85. g
18. a	52. a	86. f
19. d	53. b	87. b
20. b	54. a	88. a
21. c	55. c	89. g
22. a	56. a	90. c
23. b	57. d	91. a or l
24. b	58. b	92. d
25. a	59. c	93. b
26. a	60. d	94. f or h
27. b	61. a	95. k
28. a	62. c	96. l or a
29. c	63. a	97. i
30. b	64. e	98. h or f
31. c	65. a	99. e
32. c	66. d	100. j
33. b	67. b	
34. d	68. b	

Mission 13 Debriefing Answers

1. a	35. a	69. a
2. c	36. a	70. d
3. h	37. d	71. a
4. b	38. c	72. d
5. a	39. b	73. a
6. b	40. b	74. b
7. d	41. b	75. c
8. b	42. a	76. b
9. a	43. c	77. l
10. b	44. b	78. e
11. a	45. d	79. f
12. b	46. a	80. a
13. d	47. a	81. k
14. a	48. b	82. d
15. b	49. d	83. g
16. d	50. b	84. b
17. c	51. d	85. j
18. b	52. c	86. h
19. b	53. a	87. c
20. b	54. d	88. i
21. b	55. d	89. i
22. c	56. b	90. g
23. c	57. a	91. h
24. d	58. c	92. l
25. b	59. a	93. j
26. a	60. b	94. d
27. b	61. c	95. e
28. b	62. d	96. f
29. c	63. d	97. a or k
30. b	64. b	98. k or a
31. c	65. b	99. c
32. b	66. b	100. b
33. e	67. a	
34. a	68. h	

Bibliography of Helpful Works

Blumberg, Marvin A. (1998) HFC-170, Updated: 06/30/2010. Information on Importation of Drugs Prepared by the Division of Import Operations and Policy, FDA Retrieved from: http://www.fda.gov/ForIndustry/ImportProgram/ucm173751.htm

Class II Type B2 Laminar Flow Biological Safety Cabinets at Ordering Criteria for the National Institutes of Health (2010) Retrieved from: http://www.ors.od.nih.gov/sr/dohs/Documents/B2_BSC_Specifications.pdf

Dib, Jean G, Abdulmohsin, Saud A, Farooki, Masood U, Mohammed, Khurram, Iqbal, Mohammed, and Khan, Jamal Ahmed. (2006). Effects of an Automated Drug Dispensing System on Medication Adverse Event Occurrences and Cost Containment at SAMSO. *Hospital Pharmacy*, 41(12) 1180–1184. Retrieved from: http://www.factsandcomparisons.com/assets/hpdatenamed/20061201_dec2006_peer2.pdf

Drug Facts and Comparisons. (2011) St. Louis: Facts and Comparisons

Electronic Health Records Page. last Modified: 03/26/2012 3:42 PM
http://www.cms.gov/Medicare/E-Health/EHealthRecords/index.html?redirect=/EHealthRecords

EHR Incentive Programs. Page last Modified: 05/01/2012 1:27 PM
http://www.cms.gov/Regulations-and-Guidance/Legislation/EHRIncentivePrograms/index.html

Evans, Mary E and Barry S. Reiss.(1990). *Pharmacological Aspects of Nursing Care*. New York: Delmar Publishers

Garcia, Daniel E and Liz Johnson Wilroy. (2002).*Pharmacy Sterile Products Training Manual*. Houston: Pharmacy Education Resources, Inc

Guidance for Industry Sterile Drug Products Produced by Aseptic Processing — Current Good Manufacturing Practice. (2004). Retrieved from: http://www.fda.gov/downloads/Drugs/GuidanceComplianceRegulatoryInformation/Guidances/ucm070342.pdf

Grandics, Peter. (2000). Pyrogens and Parenteral Pharmaceuticals. *Pharmaceutical Technology*
Retrieved from: http://cypress-international.com/image/sterogene/endotoxin.html

Hunt, Max L, Jr. *Training Manual for Intravenous Admixture Personnel*. (1995).Chicago: Precept Press/Baxter Healthcare Corporation

LoBuono, Charlotte. (2007). Hospital pharmacies to go high-tech and decentralized. *Drug Topics*
Health-System Edition Retrieved from: http://drugtopics.modernmedicine.com/drugtopics/Special+Reports/Hospital-pharmacies-to-go-high-tech-and-decentrali/ArticleStandard/Article/detail/411521

Making Health Care Safer: A Critical Analysis of Patient Safety Practices. Evidence Report/Technology Assessment, No. 43. AHRQ Publication No. 01-E058, July 2001. Agency for Healthcare Research and Quality, Rockville, MD. Retrieved from: http://www.ahrq.gov/clinic/ptsafety

Pyrogens, Still a Danger. Updated: 06/16/2010
Retrieved from: http://www.fda.gov/iceci/inspections/inspectionguides/inspectiontechnicalguides/ucm072906.htm

Polin, Jenevieve Blair. (2002). Alternatives to PVC for IV Bags. *Pharmaceutical and Medical Packaging News*. Retrieved from:
http://www.pmpnews.com/article/alternatives-pvc-iv-bags

McCann, Milenkovic L. (1992). Effects of thymosin alpha-1 on pituitary hormone release. Neuroendocrinology. 55(1):14-9. Retrieved from:
http://www.ncbi.nlm.nih.gov/pubmed/1319003

Mosher, William D and Jones, Jo.(2010). Use of Contraception in the United States: 1982–2008. Retrieved from:
http://www.cdc.gov/nchs/data/series/sr_23/sr23_029.pdf

Rajfer, Jacob, (2000). Relationship Between Testosterone and Erectile Dysfunction, Reviews in Urology 2(2). Retrieved from:
http://www.ncbi.nlm.nih.gov/pmc/articles/PMC1476110/

Roman Numerals 101 Course. Retrieved from: www.oliverlawrence.com/romans101

The Human Body, *World Book Encyclopedia of Science, Volume 7*.(1992)Chicago: World Book, Inc.

Workers' Rights.(n.d.). Retrieved from: http://www.osha.gov/Publications/osha3021.pdf

www.cdc.gov
www.dea.gov
www.drugs.com/top200.html
www.drugstore.com
www.fda.gov
www.heart.org
www.jcaho.org
www.labconco.com
www.nabp.net
www.osha.gov
www.pharmlabs.unc.edu/labs
www.rxlist.com
www.rxlist.com/script/main/hp.asp
www.who.int

CPSIA information can be obtained
at www.ICGtesting.com
Printed in the USA
BVOW04s2018310817

493392BV00025B/170/P